MYSTICAL MEDICINE

By
Warren R. Peters

TEACH Services, Inc.
Brushton, New York

Copyright © 1995 TEACH Services, Inc.

ISBN 1-57258-044-5
Library of Congress Catalog Card No. 95-61242

Published by

TEACH Services, Inc.
Route 1, Box 182
Brushton, New York 12916

INTRODUCTION

This book was written as a documentation of my personal quest for a truthful knowledge of healing. The search led into broad and varied pathways-history, mythology, psychology, spiritualism, modern and ancient medicine, and religion. It was a trip I needed to take, far beyond my normal boundaries of technical medicine.

While I do not expect all readers to agree with every conclusion that I draw, I would ask that we each look at this material honestly. Do not take the references to your healing philosophy personally, but instead look at the origins and roots of each method of healing. To truly understand healing, we must go far beyond the superficial evaluation.

In the final analysis, this is a spiritual book. The Scriptures tell us that "spiritual things are spiritually discerned." Therefore, I invite you to ask God to open your mind to His reality. This world is indeed involved in a "great controversy." And even though the outcome has grave cosmic ramifications, the battle is being fought on the soil of our minds. That is why I urge you to read this book prayerfully.

Warren R. Peters, M.D.

ACKNOWLEDGMENTS

A book which has lingered in the development stages can become frustrating. However, there are many advantages as well. A special note of thanks must go to those many people who have read the book in manuscript and have given their honest and faithful criticism. The many questions that have been raised by those listening to my lectures on this topic have stimulated me to dig deeper, and there is still much to learn. I want to particularly thank Donna Harley, Kathy Goley, Cheryl Grams, Linda Ball and our untiring Health Science students who did the final editing. Wives who become "computer widows" deserve special commendation, and Jeanne is no exception. Without her support and understanding, this book would not have become a reality. Finally, I want to thank the Holy Spirit for patiently listening to my pleas for help to articulate my findings accurately in written form. May God be praised!

CONTENTS

Chapter One

THE REVELATION

Today many people are becoming aware of the relationship that exists between the mind, body, and spirit for achieving total health. As a Christian physician with many years of traditional, humanistic, medical and surgical training, I began to awaken to the concept of the "whole man." I started to study books authored by Hans Selye, M.D., Nathan Pritikin, O. Carl Simonton, M.D., René Dubos, Norman Cousins and James Lynch. I even "dabbled" for the first time into Christian books like *Ministry of Healing* and *Medical Ministry.* I perceived a common thread of world brotherhood and mind expansion which could solve the tension I felt in my materialistic and technocratic surgical world. Perhaps the practice of surgery did hold more challenge than just another bypass operation which, I knew from experience, merely postponed death, but did little to change the cause of the underlying disease condition.

I became interested in the popular holistic health movement as it began to sweep over this country. It was gratifying and reassuring to see that practitioners of the "holistic arts" were concerned about the totality of man, and I felt a certain camaraderie with them. Frustration in my own field gave way to hope for a better, more humane method of practice. It was rather stimulating to be on the edge of "new frontiers" in medicine. It was exhilarating to be a medical heretic, and challenge the stuffy "medical establishment." There was a delightful informality with these practitioners. We hugged each other and accepted one another with our various peculiarities. This openness among the holistic professionals was in marked contrast to the highly competitive, formal atmosphere of traditional medicine. We had common goals in the lifestyle areas of nutrition and exercise. We even talked about the spiritual aspects of man, something that was strictly forbidden in the standard practice of medicine. "Leave those matters to the clergy and get on with the technology of saving lives," was the implied directive from modern allopathic medicine. But for what reason? There had to be more to life than the latest technical advances in synthetic arteries or woven Dacron prosthetic grafts. What was happening to the "souls" and "spirits" of the human beings who were receiving those synthetic arteries? Who was taking care of their tears and hurts? Who cared about the whole person?

One evening I was asked to speak at a local holistic health meeting that met in the pleasant, comfortable home of several health professionals. There was much expression of acceptance and love. No one was ignored and I immediately felt at ease. As the meeting began, we were led in an exercise of "centering" by a large, soft-spoken man. His melodious voice called us to lay aside the hectic activities of the day and to "become focused" on our immediate surroundings and on one another's personal needs. We were to empty our minds of any negative thoughts and to become open to any ideas that would flow through our discussion. We quietly closed our eyes, relaxed, and centered our attention on each other and the "rhythm of life." Because of my Christian social upbringing, I thought we were just having "opening prayer." There were some rather vague references to a "unified consciousness" which, in my naivety, I assumed referred to God. This idea made me feel even more at ease with this "family" of nurses, doctors, and research scientists. This was certainly no wild-eyed "hippie" group. They were "caring" professionals that I could trust. That night I spoke to them about vegetarianism and its impact on health. The topic was well received and many expressed interest in the fact that my church heritage included healthful teaching. Even though my Christian church ties were quite weak at that point, I felt like a real missionary. These people were accepting of all beliefs, including Christian, Hindu, Buddhist, Jewish, and atheist.

The next speaker was a registered nurse from a local hospital cardiac care unit. With convincing organization and well thought-out conclusions, she presented the concepts of "touch therapy." Without actually touching the patient's body, the practitioner could purportedly adjust his "electrical aura." This adjustment was accomplished by allowing the hands to flow above the limbs and trunk with spiral movements. We divided into groups of two's and practiced our "innate" ability to sense the "vibrations" of energy that she had said "clothed" the body. I wasn't sure that I could truly sense what she described or what my partner enthusiastically experienced, but then, maybe I just needed more practice. I could feel the warmth of her skin next to mine. Thermal radiation I could explain physiologically, but this was supposed to be something different. Perhaps there was "energy" of which I was not fully aware.

The nurse then had a doctor lie down on the floor while she moved "congested energy" from his pelvic region to his legs. The doctor was able to testify that he indeed experienced a strange, but comfortable tingling and warmth in his lower extremities. As a peripheral vascular surgeon, this assertion was of great interest to me. I was thinking about this new "energy" and how it could be used to save those gangrenous legs and toes in cases where bypass is impossible and amputation is the only sad solution. It certainly sounded more "natural" and humane than amputation. My mind was focused on those pathetic people that I longed to help, and often could not. Perhaps this was the help that scientific advances had been unable to supply.

The nurse then moved her hands over the physician's chest in the same circular pattern. Suddenly she stopped and with a cry of exclamation said, "You have a hard time completing tasks, don't you?" I was jolted to reality. The soft lights and pleasant voices no longer clouded my thinking. What had I heard? Was she "divining" his personality characteristics from these supposed "vibrations"?

The situation I was dealing with suddenly became clear. This experience opened my mind to the realization that I must investigate the origin and mode of operation of these phenomena. This was not some simple physiological technique that modern medicine had overlooked. Instead, it seemed to be a tool of "divining" the future. What did Scripture say about the power of Satan? Could he be the source of these "good techniques"?

> The coming of the lawless one will be in accordance with the work of Satan, displayed in all kinds of counterfeit miracles, signs and wonders, and in every sort of evil that deceives those who are perishing. They perish because they refuse to love the truth and so be saved.[1]

This is the great controversy. Satan can and will do miracles. After His resurrection, Jesus was triumphantly taken from His disciples, victorious over His archenemy. We are told that

> Satan again counseled with his angels, and with bitter hatred against God's government, told them that while he retained his power and authority upon earth, their efforts must be tenfold stronger against the followers of Jesus. They had prevailed nothing against Christ, but must overthrow His followers, if possible.[2]

Satan is using any and every method to snare the followers of Christ. I believe that the medical movement called "holistic health" is a part of Satan's master plan to capture unwary, yet well-meaning people. Many, such as I, have read a smattering of inspired writings about health, and have a shallow understanding of the Scriptures, but have never really taken the time to systematically decipher what God is really trying to tell Christians about the health of mind, body, and spirit. Armed with a few selected quotations from "religious" writers and Scripture texts that tend to "prove" the validity of their "pet therapy" or technique, well-meaning Christians have jumped wholeheartedly into this movement.

Where did holistic medicine come from? Where does it lead? These questions bothered me and I determined to investigate them. My study led me back, far back into history.

Chapter Two

THE WAY IS PREPARED

In scanning the misty horizons of history, there emerges a definite pattern of cycles. History repeats itself. Even heresies of ages past are re-expressed in the next age with new words of excitement and intellectual intrigue, effectively camouflaging the same old satanic sophistries.

The century prior to the French Revolution was filled with the formalization of religion. Great cathedrals of splendor were common in every city and hamlet of Europe. Large numbers of priests and members of the clerical hierarchy enjoyed positions of honor and support within the governmental structure. It was in this system, and with great piety and pretense, that the papal powers slaughtered thousands of faithful Christian believers. Personal Christian piety was not present among the ruling clerics. Instead, immorality, debauchery, and theft dominated the lives of these "men and women of God." The ordinary person experienced a declining level of respect for the church and its leadership, but fear and ignorance often kept him in stifled submission to a degenerate system of church.

The Holy Scriptures were removed from general use, and locked up with the claim that they were too holy to be observed or studied by the common man on the street. This concept was consistent with the social structure of the times, in which the masses of working people were despised and exploited by the privileged few who formed the religious hierarchy. The uplifting influence of the Bible was lost, in fulfillment of that which was foretold in the Scriptures.

And I will give power to my two witnesses, and they prophe-
sied for 1,260 days, clothed in sackcloth…. Now when they
have finished their testimony, the beast that comes up from
the abyss will attack them, and overpower and kill them.
Their bodies will lie in the street of the great city, which is
figuratively called Sodom and Egypt, where also their Lord
was crucified.[1]

These "two witnesses," the Old and the New Testaments,
were almost completely and effectively destroyed. In fact, in
France, they were officially denounced. "The world for the first
time heard an assembly of men, born and educated in civilization, and assuming the right to govern one of the finest of the
European nations, uplift their united voice to deny the most
solemn truth which man's soul receives, and renounce unani-
mously the belief and worship of a Deity."[2]

…but France stands apart in the world's history as the single
state which, by the decree of her Legislative Assembly,
pronounced that there was no God, and of which the entire
population of the capital, and a vast majority elsewhere,
women as well as men, danced and sang with joy in accep-
tancy of the announcement.[3]

Into this vacuum entered the "Intellectual Revolution."

To Descartes, the physical universe appeared to be a vast
machine created by a supreme mathematician. "The laws of
nature are identical with the laws of mechanics," he declared.
"You can substitute the mathematical order of the universe
for God whenever I use the latter term."[4]

With the rise of natural philosophy, theology was displaced
from its proud position as "Queen of the Sciences." The
Great Schism, the Revival of Learning, and the Protestant
Reformation had all tended to weaken the unity and authority
of the medieval church…. By the eighteenth century, religious fervor was yielding its spirit to tolerance and indiffer-
ence…. Some skeptics dared to repudiate all belief in an
Infinite Power and to deny that the theologians were or ever
had been the custodians of Divine truths which could guide

7

men to salvation.... The new learning allowed man to see himself as independent. This bolstered his pride, whereas his religious beliefs had fruited in humility.... But the rationalists had moved to question this view. "Perhaps," they suggested, "man was intended to control his own destiny, instead of bowing fatalistically to the will of an inscrutable Providence...." They preferred to conceive of God as a remote and impersonal deity, a First Cause of First Principle, or an ideal constitutional monarch who never violated the laws which He had established for the government of the natural realm.[5]

With the first blush of this newfound scientific thought came the hope that man could solve many of the dilemmas of the world by more intensive research into "natural law." There seemed to be less need for the supernatural or a "power outside of ourselves." In fact, there was very little need for God at all. Since in their minds He had been previously associated with the oppressive and unprogressive stupefying clergy, the "rational man" was glad to be free from God. Man could now progress without God, using his own materials and resources to make his world a better place.

Magnetism and electricity and their mysterious intangibility intrigued this generation of scientists. Before, natural things had been limited to the "material"—things that could be seen and touched. But now, energy, once seen as separate from substantial matter, was thought to be the very "essence" of material things. Electricity and the magnet could be felt, and its effects studied, but it could not be seen. Man was pushing the "frontiers" of science. Speculation about the heavenly bodies revived in the context of magnetism and electricity. The ancient attraction to celestial study and its effect on human life once again became generally popular. This was unknown territory. Electricity was now going to answer questions and unlock power that the church or gods could never have answered or given.

We have just witnessed, in retrospect, a pattern of history as it emerges, only to be repeated in different forms in different ages to come. First comes a religious decline, and then the development of materialism fueled by scientific advances. The scientific progress is seen as the solution to all social and material woes—the answer that will end all questions. But there is a flaw in this logic. Materialism and science, no matter how pompous and prestigious, can never meet the needs of the inner spiritual nature of man. The great questions still arise, "Where have we come from and what is going to happen to us when we die?"

In the late eighteenth and early nineteenth centuries, man once again began to look for spiritual answers. God's name had been dragged in the dirt by the clergy of the day, and the materialistic, rational man had denied His existence. here, an important fact is ignored. There are only two powers in the universe: God and Satan. And unfortunately, if the existence of God has been ruled out, then the spiritual questions get satanic answers by default.

During this same time, there was in Europe and America an amazing rebirth of Spiritualism, which took on many faces. With the existing interest in magnetism and astronomy, Satan was able to use these methods to deceive mankind. He has never been deficient in finding new disguises for error, and doltishly, man accepts even his "redressed" ancient sophistries.

> Franz Anton Mesmer, of Suabia, came to Vienna to study medicine under van Swieten and de Haem. His graduating thesis, "The Influence of the Planets in the Cure of Diseases" (1766), promulgated the theory that the sun and moon act upon living beings by means of the subtle fluid known as animal magnetism, analogous in its effect to the properties of the lodestone. Mesmer thus revealed himself as a belated medical astrologer, a congenital mystic. He claimed he could magnetize trees so that every leaf contributed healing to all who approached.[6]

Mesmer gained notoriety for his temple to the god of health. Patients from all parts of Europe entered those halls of incense and ethereal music, searching expectantly for "healing." Mesmer had forsaken his former ideas of impersonal magnetism for something more "natural." He and other male "practitioners" now replaced the lodestone and magnetic coils. They were the magnets!

> The patients sat around a magnetic "bequet" [tub], and waited. The majority were women, and for them a special set of handsome young men had been provided. Slowly and solemnly these assistant magnetizers marched forward and each selected a woman and stared her in the eyes. No words were spoken, but from somewhere softly sailed the music of an accordion, and the voice of a hidden opera-singer sweetened the incense laden air. The young Apollos embraced the knees of the women, rubbed various spots, and gently massaged their breasts. The women closed their eyes, and felt the magnetism surge through them. At the critical moment, the master magnetizer, Mesmer himself, appeared on the scene. Clad in a lilac gown, with lofty mien and majestic tread, he advanced among his patients, making "passes" and accomplishing miracles.[7]

Lest he be thought to be an obscure "alternative practitioner," we should note that the French government offered Anton Mesmer a pension and the Cross of the Order of St. Michael, if he would divulge his secret. He was making a fortune and refused the pension. He might have done well to accept the offer, however, because later his practice was investigated by a group of illustrious scientists of the eighteenth century, including Benjamin Franklin and Lavoisier, who did not accept the spiritual concepts and consequences of this technique. They explained away the whole thing as a fraud based on the "imagination."

The idea of "animal magnetism" was at first ridiculed by James Braid, (1795–1861), a surgeon of Fifeshire, Scotland, "but he soon became convinced, upon experimentation, that there can be a genuine self-induced sleep brought about by a fixed stare at a bright, inanimate object."[8] Through the influence of Dr. Braid, "animal magnetism" was given scientific credibility.

Satan did not really care what "stamp" it was given. He only desired that the ensnaring technique be used by human beings to the destruction of their souls.

Germany was also affected by the subjective mystical forms of therapy. History reveals to us that Europe was so intellectually and morally exhausted by the Napoleonic wars, that the way was prepared for the wildest kind of speculation.[9] It was not only "animal magnetism" that was sweeping Europe, but also odic force [all substances radiate an omnipresent force as experienced by psychics], homeopathy, phrenology, and sympathetic medicine including "stroking" or "touch therapy."

In stark contrast, some Christians of the New World were becoming interested in health and a natural lifestyle. Oberlin College, a prominent Christian institution in Ohio, adopted a largely vegetarian diet. Tea and coffee were not served, and exercise in the out-of-doors was promoted. Williams College, Hudson College, and Lane Seminary all followed an awakening interest in health. The Seventh-day Adventist Church, arising from the religious awakening of the 1840's, took a strong stand against the "drugging business" of standard medical practice. Instead of arsenic, mercury, bleeding, and other harmful practices, these Christians advocated a radical separation from the medical "orthodoxy" of that day and espoused the use of exercise, diet, sunlight and simple water therapies for the preservation of health. This Christian church also took a strong stand against the spiritualistic methods of Europe.

> Thousands, I was shown, have been spoiled through the philosophy of phrenology and animal magnetism, and have been driven into infidelity. If the mind commences to run in this channel, it is almost sure to lose its balance and be controlled by a demon.[10]

The origin of such methodology is not left open to question.

> They are venturing on the devil's ground and are tempting him to control them. This powerful destroyer considers them his lawful prey, exercising his power upon them, and that against their will. When they wish to control themselves, they cannot. They yielded their minds to Satan, and he will not release his claims, but holds them captive. No power can deliver the ensnared soul but the power of God in answer to the earnest prayers of His faithful followers.[11]

Why then did Spiritualism gain a foothold in America during the mid-eighteen hundreds? And why do we find spiritualistic teaching invading and pervading our soil again by way of the holistic health and New Age movement?

Chapter Three

NEW AGE SUCCESS

Jonah slept while the storm tore at the ship. The wind and waves thrashed the tiny wooden vessel. The veteran sailors were terrified and frantically began doing what they could to survive. How could Jonah sleep now, while the very lives of all aboard were threatened? He was, indeed, in a DEEP SLEEP! When God has given an assignment that is deliberately ignored, only deep sleep will be sufficient to cover a smarting conscience. God chose a pagan sea captain to awaken Jonah. Jonah had to be physically shaken and a penetrating question and command put to him to awaken him from his stuporous sleep. "How can you sleep? Get up and call on your God! Maybe He will take notice of us, and we will not perish."[1]

The Christian church has been given a commission to warn a world on the brink of the impending Apocalypse. A deep sleep permeates our very being. The world is lashed and torn, but we sleep on with the message of security and peace locked within our minds. Oh, it is true that we are on our way to "the world," but not to warn it! No! that would be too invasive. Instead we are on our way to becoming like the world. We want to be a good "influence" in the world rather than warning the world. Perhaps a public relations spree would depict us as "caring people." But certainly, let us not sound like alarmists. The Christian community has not effectively addressed the dehumanization of man by technology, and the deep hurt of mankind bound by

> Eastern metaphysics and the New Consciousness, on the other hand, derive their popularity in part from the fact that

they directly challenge the oppressive assumptions of the technocratic Western mentality.

destroying habits. Yes, confession can be heard from the pulpit, but is there any POWER available that can change our faulty thinking patterns and death-dealing lifestyle? Can real PERSONHOOD be found while standing eight hours a day in a boring and dehumanizing production line of machines? Am I important or valuable to the universe?

Without God-centered answers to these questions, a deep void has been created by generations of horrible atrocities. A nation of churchgoing people attempted to destroy from the face of the earth a single ethnic group of humans. A nation with its coinage reading "In God We Trust," developed and deployed an atomic blast that instantly destroyed men, women, and children who innocently belonged to a race who was at war. The void was deepened by industrial nations which began to develop by-products that poisoned the very atmosphere and polluted precious water supplies. Was there a Christian outcry? No! It all kept happening and sweet little people continued playing church, ignoring the poor, ignoring the disadvantaged, establishing another impersonal, inefficient agency to care for them. The personal and social void is now monstrously deep.

Into this void stepped the New Age movement. Its adherents are tireless. They will work, give, and share day or night. Pay, hours, and benefits are not their motives. They embrace all businesses, governments, and religious persuasions, and offer a "solution" to the personal and social voids of the day. They do believe in what they are doing. There is a religious fervor to the approach and attitude of the New Age or "New Consciousness" person. Because of the narrow perspective of materialism, life in general has not met the inherent spiritual needs of mankind. In contrast, the New Age offers a blend of humanism linked with a strong, eclectic, spiritual enthusiasm. Pantheism, Monism, Spiritualism, Hinduism and many others "isms" have been liberally mixed into this caldron of deception.

14

And the church sleeps on! Perhaps no one has depicted this phenomenon more clearly than David Fetcho:

> They have not been afraid to charge our rationalist, materialist, mercantile culture with depleting the quality of human life. They have suggested that our 'normal' way of looking at things is deficient at best. Leaders of New Age movements have stepped into the vacancy created by the silence of the church. They call plastic plastic and poison poison in a society whose economy is built on convincing people that both are good for them.... They have taken the lead in demonstrating the possibility of changing from a denatured diet to an organic one, from an ethic of consumerism to one of economic simplicity, from big business, profit-oriented medicine to individualized healing of the whole person and preventive health care. From drugged childbirth and carcinogenic baby foods, to natural childbirth and a dedication to wholesome child rearing.[2]

In the 1940's, a man began to write from the concentration camps of Germany. He asked earnest questions and sought answers that fit the reality of war, filth and hate. Dietrich Bonhoeffer's writings conceived a "Christianity without religion." It substituted daily life, or "reality," for a caring, personal God. This concept, which he chose to call "ground of all being," was his attempt to somehow bring "God" to those who did not "need" God. To Bonhoeffer, the "human encounter" was the only

hope of "reality." His attempts to bring a spiritual dimension to plain old humanism completely destroyed the supernatural, Biblical concept of spiritual creation and re-creation.

In 1949, Paul Tillich wrote the book *The Shaking of the Foundation,* which redefined even the basic words of Christianity.

> The name of this infinite and inexhaustible depth and ground of all being is God. That depth is what the word 'God' means. And if that word has not much meaning for you, translate it, and speak of the depths of your life, of the source

of your being, of your ultimate concern, of what you take seriously without any reservation.[3]

In *Honest to God,* John A. T. Robinson, an Anglican bishop, attempts to respond to the God "up there" or "out there," and the dilemma caused by the absence of God's personal involvement in "real life" as he perceives it. These sincere efforts to harmonize the rise of materialism did not cause the "God-is-dead" movement, but only signaled the fact that it had already happened. Man saw his "God" as irrelevant and impotent. It seems strange that it did not occur to these men that it was not God who had died, but instead, their connection to Him had been willfully severed. When God is not seen as the active Creator and Sustainer of life, there is little left to the concept of God and religion. Man, "come of age" as Dr. Robinson would say, can only see human relationships as a source of "spiritual" fulfillment. By his reasoning, mature human beings do not need the God of Biblical interpretation. A God such as that would be only for the weak and immature.[4]

With this loss of true piety, religion first becomes formalized, then depersonalized, and finally, humanistic terms are given to everything that God does. Now "God" is not only absent "in me," but He is no longer "out there" or "up there"! This creates a dilemma since a "God" concept has always been active and vital in the history of mankind. Therefore, the only hope of both the disillusioned cleric and the Eastern mystic is to develop a "God" of his own making.

Paul Tillich, in commenting on the majestic 139th Psalm of David, says,

> There is no ultimate privacy or final isolation. We are always held and comprehended by something that is greater than we are, that has a claim upon us, and that demands response from us. The most intimate motions within the depths of our souls are not completely our own, for they belong also to our friends, to mankind, to the universe, and to the ground of all being, the aim of our life…. Omnipresence means that our privacy is public. The center of our whole being is involved

in the center of all being: and the center of all being rests in the center of our being.[5]

Now compare a bit of "New Age" theology by Werner Erhard, founder of EST (Erhard Seminars Training). "The Self itself is the 'ground of all being,' that from which everything arises."[6] "When I get in touch with myself and you get in touch with yourself, we will see the same self."[7]

To our amazement, we find that the theology of Tillich and the New Age thinking of Erhard have their roots in ancient Buddhism. Such thinking is expressed in the following commentary on Zen Buddhism. "In the higher realm of True Suchness there is neither 'other' nor 'self.' When a direct identification is asked for, we can only say, 'Not two.' One in all, all in one—if only this is realized, no more worry about your not being perfect!"[8] This Monistic thinking, in which there is no individual, but each is part of the cosmic whole, reduces life to a subjective mass of individual interpretation. As Erhard would say, "If you did it, it must be good." This reasoning justifies murder, theft, child abuse, and rape. When Christianity refuses to play the strong role of world guide, the vacuum is quickly filled by the subtle delusions of spiritualized humanism. Man is even defined in God-like terms. The Creator is lost sight of, as the creature assumes the role of his own deity.

It is now time, yes, past time, for the church to awaken from its slumber. Let us not rant against the New Age movement when in reality its existence is only a symptom of our deep coma. "If once we catch a glimpse of that glorious vision, perhaps then we may abandon our futile journey to Tarshish, and find, with Jonah, that acceptance of the judgment of God is acceptance of His grace."[9]

Chapter Four

THE TECHNIQUES

In the previous chapters, we have looked briefly at the general philosophical background and the rise of the New Age movement in America today. Within this movement can be found "holistic health," a diverse collection of healing techniques. We must have a thorough understanding of the origin and details of some of these methods.

> All who do not earnestly search the Scriptures and submit every desire and purpose of life to that unerring test, all who do not seek God in prayer for a knowledge of His will, will surely wander from the right path and fall under the deception of Satan.... His agents still claim to cure disease. They attribute their power to electricity, magnetism, or the so-called 'sympathetic remedies.' In truth, they are but channels for Satan's electric currents. By this means he casts his spell over the bodies and souls of men.[1]

No quotation has captured my attention more than this succinct description of the actual techniques that Satan does use. "Satan's electric currents" are an accurate description of the "energy field" concepts which dominate holistic health thinking. By starting with the more obvious associations, I hope that the more subtle forms of this deception will be made plain.

In the book, *Intermediate Studies of the Human Aura,* Djwal Kul outlines the concept of an external "energy field" or "aura," which he believes is now being confirmed even by science.

> In recent years, through Kirlian photography and experiments with plants, scientists have postulated the theory of

the L-field as the blueprint of life and a force-field of energy which can be observed and photographed with either scientific instruments or this specialized photography which uses neither camera nor lens.... Man is on the brink of discovering the Higher Self.[2]

The "aura" is based on the theory

that every object is enveloped in a field of magnetic energy which acts as a medium for the interplay of other energies present in its immediate environment. This magnetic energy field or MEF, is composed of seven rays related to the glands of the endocrine system. The harmony and balance of every individual and the degree and quality of each of these can be ascertained by observing the aura either subjectively, as some "sensitives" are capable of doing, or objectively using a special type of glass called a Kilner screen.[3]

Immediately, we are aware that these are not physiological concepts. Instead, these phenomena are explained in subjective, metaphysical terms which require someone to be "attuned" to these powers to describe them. Even the trappings of science do not eliminate the need for a "sensitive" person to operate them. A very sophisticated piece of scientific equipment with dials, scopes and meters does not negate the fact that in this so-called "science," the operator must be more sensitive than most people. In fact, with increasing sensitivity, the operator may no longer need the instruments! Eventually, he is *Really?* able to divine the future or make diagnostic judgments without even seeing the patient. These techniques are called radiomics or psychotromics, and are not based on objective mechanisms.

The seven "rays" of the magnetic energy field are none other than the Hindu concept of "chakras" or energy focal points. While many authors try to treat the idea of the aura and chakra as some wholesome, physiological, and natural event in all humans, Djwal Kul, in an amazing ravel of Christian terms and mystical parlance, helps us to see the true origin of this idea.

MYSTICAL MEDICINE *Imagine* How subtle, the Devil!

> The seven centers in your being are for the release of God's
> energy.... These seven centers are seven planes of con-
> sciousness. We experience God differently in different fre-
> quencies.... What, then, is worthy to inherit God? Only God
> is worthy of God. Unless we sense ourselves in and AS
> GOD, we will not consider ourselves to be worthy of God.
> Therefore, that which inherits immortal life is the immortal
> flow of God which we make our own through the chakras.[4]
> (emphasis supplied) THE NERVE! Blasphemous!

How could we be God?

The human being, the creature of God, has now, in the height
of blasphemous audacity, taken the omniscience of God and
claimed it as his own. This creates an ever-ascending sequence
of power which is related to the pyramid in form and philosophy. Even though the "heart chakra" is the most important, and
the "throat chakra" is the center for energy control, it is the
"crown chakra" that allows the control of time and space and
"knowing all things." The spiral is the recurring geometric
design that is used to illustrate the progression toward "god-
hood." To those who hold to the theory of auras and chakras,
this assumption of God's power would cause little concern
because to them there is no God, except the god developed
within their own consciousness.

Before leaving this study of the geometry of the aura, it is
important to recognize its kinship to the symbol of medical care
today. Here we find another spiral, consisting of "the four
petals forming the base of the figure-eight pattern—even the
flow of the caduceus—that crosses in the heart of man and
reaches its culmination in the crown of life.... White light
bursts forth as a thousand suns signal across the skies the
fohatic emanations of the eternal Logos."[5] The symbol of the
"cross" and the "caduceus" are intertwined. The caduceus has
been seen in the Western world as the symbol of healing, but,
sadly, it is deeply embedded in paganism and mythology. Asclepius was a god of healing who carried a knotted staff or
cross upon which coiled a serpent. The cross on which our
wonderful Jesus was crucified was a hateful symbol of Satan-

ism, thus making this form of death even more appalling and humiliating to our Saviour. The occultic symbol of the serpent is also intertwined with the immoral pagan phallic cults. The cross and the serpent are symbols that are used to visualize the occult philosophy of chakras and auras, which are also brought into this form of self-worship.

The seven chakras have each been assigned a specific color—one of the seven "natural" colors-red-orange-yellow, green, turquoise-blue, and violet. These colors form the basis for color therapy, another of Satan's medical, diagnostic, and therapeutic schemes. Even though it is true that certain colors look better on one individual or another, and that some colors are "warm" or "cool," color therapy itself is deeply embedded in spiritism. By adding an eighth color, magenta, color therapy creates an octave which makes it possible to add music to the therapy plan. Even spinal therapy can harmonize with that system since there are twenty-four vertebrae. The twenty-four Zodiac signs can be used also. Thus is created an extension of the chakras or aura to colors, music, chiropractics, and the Zodiac. "There are three basic ways in which color therapy can be applied: (a) through colored fabrics, walls and illumination, (b) by mental image making, counseling and guided meditation, and (c) through projection, on the spiritual level, to any person anywhere."[6] These methods and techniques seem to be harmless to the average person, but in reality, participation places the person within Satan's grasp. He becomes desensitized to further steps in the downward path.

"Gem therapy" is yet another branch of the aura theory. Various stones have been correlated with the signs of the Zodiac, numerology, colors, and the chakras. After a medium has ascertained the proper gem treatment for "increased energy," the stone can be either worn on the person, hung in the workplace or placed in the drinking water. Crystals are of particular value in this occult art. Thus, it is surprising to see crystals hanging in the windows of Christian homes and cars. The practice of gem therapy is very ancient, and it is the basis of jewelry and ornamentation. To the unwitting, the crystal prism may seem very harmless and "pretty," but it can be an open door for Satan's influence. I have personally seen the practitioners of the "art" demonstrate to an audience the "energy" of gems with an electronic "divining rod" or "witch stick" The use of the "divining rod" for this occult practice is no different from its use in the discovery of water, minerals or oil.—(See chapter five)

The principles typified by the aura must be clearly understood by the reader because they will form the basis of our exploration of other holistic health techniques. First, the theory envisions an external energy force. It is important to make a distinction between this external force and the true electrical impulses of the nervous system. To be sure, each anatomical nerve carries from axon to dendrite measurable electrical current, which can be detected by any human being with standard electrical equipment. It is also true that every cell has an electrical spin, a concept that is now forming the basis of diagnostic techniques. Neither of these is an "aura." The practitioners of mystical healing methods use the aura to demonstrate external energy, which they believe is affected by thoughts and internal health. In addition, it can be seen only by those that are initiates or who are "naturally sensitive" or mediumistic.

Second, there is a distinct spiritual quality to the aura and its study. Monistic thought forms the basis for this spiritual quality in which there is no distinct, separate God. Instead, one is all and all is one. We have heard this same dictum from both the modem "God is dead" clergyman and the ancient Hindu.

In subsequent chapters, we will see these "threads" of thought woven through other techniques.

Chapter Five

THE PENDULUM AND THE STICK

After solemnly reading from Scripture the words of Christ, "Again, I tell you that if two of you on earth agree about any thing you ask for, it will be done for you by my Father in heaven," the Christian healer bowed her head in sincere prayer. Then she carefully lifted the pendulum over the sick neighbor and began to divine for the proper herb to be used for healing. If the pendulum swung clockwise, licorice root should be used, and if it swung counterclockwise, gooseberry bark would be the treatment of choice. The neighbor's eyes filled with tears of appreciation and amazement as she saw the pendulum move in various directions as questions were directed to it. She had tried several traditional doctors who had not found the cause of her illness and had only suggested side effect ridden drugs to treat her symptoms. The use of the pendulum seemed so simple and the herbs so natural, and the sweet sincerity of her Christian neighbor was so reassuring. She felt better already.

The use of the pendulum for the diagnosis and treatment of human illness is an ancient art of divination based on a concept of "unified energies." To achieve credibility and understanding, the proponents of this method explain that the body has an energy field that can be disturbed by illness. The pendulum responds to this disturbance by swinging within the magnetic field thus produced. Homeopathic medicines may also be tested by this method to determine if they would be helpful to the patient. This line of reasoning is a companion to the explanation of auras and chakras that we have already studied.

23

The pendulum may be any weight tied to a string; even a machinist's nut will work. It may be used alone or in conjunction with a very sophisticated medical apparatus. The device itself is not all that important; simple or complex, it makes no difference. What is important is the presence of a "sensitive," believing and receptive person to hold the pendulum. This has been proven over and over again with one example being the most sophisticated form of this therapy, radiaesthesia. Although the device used is complete with dials, knobs and gauges, the more "sensitive" the practitioner becomes, the less the pendulum is needed!

> Radiaesthesia is, in effect, a form of psychometry, aided by mechanical apparatus. This is not always recognized but the fact remains that it is so. The mechanism used may be a simple divining rod, a pendulum, a complicated Abrams 'box,'or one of the machines used for such work under the modem title 'radiaesthesia' or 'radionics'…. It is now admitted by those who use the various types of diagnostic machines associated with radiaesthesia that for successful work it is necessary to have present a human operator of a special type…. Hence, it follows that the accuracy or inaccuracy of diagnosis by radiaesthesia will depend upon all the usual factors involved in psychic and in medical work—experience, personality, and the conscious or unconscious psychic capacities of the operator…. Since it is claimed for such treatments that 'distance makes no difference,' this in itself rules out any likelihood that the actual healing power is etheric or dense physical. Such a suggestion conflicts with all that is known of the laws governing the radiation of energy at the physical level…. What we wish to emphasize is that the diagnoses and treatments involved should be considered as psychic or extrasensory phenomena, and that the claims made as to their being based upon purely physical science and its known laws cannot be substantiated.[1]

Other mediums, such as George Delawarr, carried radionics one step further and developed photographs from a blood sample of a patient hundreds of miles away. In one case, the lifelike

24

picture of a fetus was developed from a blood sample of a mother who was 54 miles away! Even the psychics have been frustrated with the fact that their work has very little reproducibility. Delawarr admitted in 1958 that the technique was based on the personal ability of the operator himself rather than the device.[2]

The use of the pendulum has associated itself with other equally questionable practices. One of these practices is homeopathy (see chapter ten). Hahnemann, the founder of homeopathic medicine, conceived a theory of "miasms." These "toxic factors" are the results of poorly treated (presumably by orthodox drugging) infectious diseases. The "miasms" taint the body and continue to pollute future generations as well as the affected individual. Two similar infectious diseases would, in fact, cancel each other or the symptoms could "balance" and cancel one another. Scabies and tuberculosis would be an example of this reaction according to the "miasma theory."[3] Later, these concepts were expanded to include various proteins that were thought to be over or under contracted. The use of the pendulum would help balance these problems by guiding the practitioner to supplements of vitamins, minerals or herbs that would be "anti-miasmic." These concepts formed much of the basis for the "toxin" and "balance" idea that we find so prevalent in the health food industry. The more "scientifically astute" health supplement practitioner will speak in terms of RNA or DNA potions when referring to these simple proteins.[4] (The profits of the sales organizations have gone up accordingly.)

Pendulum diagnosis and radiaesthesia became popular in Europe during the early twentieth century largely because of the extraordinary ability of Abbes Mermet, a French priest. His "gift" allowed him to not only heal, but also find water, treasure and minerals. Note carefully that without leaving his house, Mermet would use the pendulum over a map and find water 6000 miles away![5]

Those that use the pendulum equate their work with "water witching." Since this form of divination is more widely accepted by the general public, it is hoped that this association will lend credibility to the use of the pendulum. Sadly, water witching has a similar sordid connection with the occult. You may want to prove this to yourself by looking through the occult section of your bookstore. Robert H. Leftwich freely admits that his knowledge and ability came through the occult.

> ...I have always been intensely interested in all forms of ESP and the occult. In an effort to increase this knowledge, I had built up quite a substantial library over the years, from which I was then able to extract much information on dowsing.[6]

From this background, Leftwich attempts to explain these strange powers that he now possesses. He is not quite ready to admit that they are evil, but acknowledges that they are definitely "subconscious supernormal cognitive faculties." Since this ability is primarily in the mind, he can at least foresee the possibility that evil could result.

> The basic characteristics of humanity have not been changed by history. Modern dowsers are completely unaware of the forces they are tapping, they do not realize the potential power at their disposal. Although invariably utilized to benefit humanity through healing and other useful means, this can just as easily be channeled along different lines to provide almost unlimited scope in many other fields, including antisocial activity. When these forces are combined with the ability to consciously create circumstances, almost all desires can be realized.[7]

I could certainly support the thesis that most dowsers do not recognize the power with which they are dealing. Those who seek healing from the pendulum or find water through the witch stick must look beyond the immediate results and see the potential of evil consequences.

To further demonstrate the pathway of witchcraft through these modalities, note the following quotation.

The fundamental concept, however, is that man possesses an etheric counterpart which under normal conscious conditions coincides with his physical body but, depending on his natural periodicity or biorhythm, this can be partially or completely projected from it. In this condition, he is frequently able to see himself as a separate entity and, after some experience, can project his ethereal body, or 'vehicle of the soul' as it is sometimes termed, quite a distance from the physical body, although he is usually very much aware of the existence of an ethereal connection between the two.[8]

Now we find ourselves dealing with "astral projection," reincarnation, and spirit bodies. Christian, how much more evidence do you need! Ben Hester's latest book, *Dowsing—An Expose' of Hidden Occult Forces* states,

We must say it again; involvement in the dowsing scene is a matter of choosing whom you will serve. The idea of choosing to dowse, as being a pact with Satan, is ridiculed by the liberal Christian as well as the non-Christian. It is a fact, nevertheless, that any involvement with the occult implies required loyalty. If these are not elements of a pact, perhaps we are only hung up on semantics.[9]

Despite evidence from the writings of witchers and their critics alike, there are those who still think that this is a "neutral" physical power that can be used either for good or evil. If it is a natural, neutral, physical phenomenon that follows the laws of nature, why do not all tree branches turn downward over water? If it is some common natural force, think what would happen if your dog was carrying a stick over an underground water source. Can you see the stick twisting in the dog's mouth? Or think of how difficult it would be to carry an arm load of branches over a creek or spring. A physical law? No, this is an occult art.

The following story of a Christian family's brush with the satanic practice of pendulum diagnosis is both instructive and revealing. After some misgivings, the father made an appointment with the herb practitioner.

She checked me all over with the pendulum. Sometimes when she was checking she would lose the ability to check, so she would grab handfuls of apricot pits and start eating them and her ability to check would return. She also did a reflexology treatment on my feet. I needed some vitamin E and manganese according to her pendulum. At this time she was using a brass button as her pendulum. Later I learned from the herb practitioner how to use vital therapy in conjunction with the pendulum.... It was at this time that my wife began having problems breathing.... I took her to be checked by the herb practitioner. She checked positive to a handful of vitamin B-6, a handful of folic acid, and a handful of manganese.... Then she had seizures. According to the pendulum, the problem was caused by the red in some cherries that she ate.... By now I guess that you can tell that we were living our lives according to the swing of our pendulum. One of the many things we did because of the pendulum was to place our clothes out in the sun on the clothesline, and on the ground in an effort to get them positive. We spaced the clothes with our pendulum as to the best place to put them.... I would separate the clothes using the pendulum to tell which clothes to wash together. Then I would do vital therapy on each wash load till the pendulum would stop rotating to indicate positive.... One of my sons, Michael, had occasional headaches. The pendulum indicated that sugar was the problem.... For one headache the pendulum indicated the problem to be the blue kleenex he had used. For another, it was the blue sock he was wearing, or the elastic in his waist band.... Unless we were away from home or had company, I checked almost everything I ate to make sure that I was eating only things that were food for me—at least according to testing with the pendulum.[10]

Thus, the pendulum controlled the entire life of this Christian family until the father became suspicious of the origin of this method of natural healing. The pendulum seemed to be working surprisingly well that Monday morning, until while driving to work

...I felt like singing of God's love, so that's what I did. A couple of songs that I especially remember singing were: 'I Would Love to Tell You What I Think of Jesus' and 'Come Thou Fount of Every Blessing.' As I was driving along singing of God's love the thought occurred to me to try using the pendulum while singing. I picked up the pendulum, held it over my hand, but it did not move. Next I held it over my lunch, still nothing—dead as a doornail. Needless to say I was shaken, and very scared.... I had my answer! I felt as if a weight had been lifted from me. I took my pendulum and threw the thing as far into the woods as I could. I've not picked one up since. I thank God every day for His protection and deliverance from the power of Satan.[11]

To this story I can only say, "Praise God for His mercy to us—foolish creatures that we are."

To support the use of the pendulum and the witch stick, it has been alleged that one of the early pioneers of the Seventh-day Adventist Church, Ellen White, supported water witching by ordering the use of it to find water for a health resort in southern California. Even though this account has been published by her grandson in the biography, *The Early Elmshaven Years,* the veracity of this sketchy account has been thoroughly researched by Ben Hester, who is not a member of this Christian church. A comprehensive study of all the letters and writings from Ellen White during this episode has led Mr. Hester to conclude that Ellen White was not aware that water witching was being done. She was not present at that well site during the digging, and there is no evidence that she condoned or condemned the practice of water witching.[12] The absence of a condemnation of water witching certainly does not constitute an endorsement of this practice. Neither did she condemn the use of the Ouija Board, even though her many statements against spiritism would leave no doubt as to her position on the matter.

The Christian church has condemned the practice of divination since its recorded history. In 1518, Martin Luther called dowsing "the work of the Devil." This position was largely taken from the Old Testament statement that clearly spoke against the use of a "wooden staff" for divination.[13] I believe that John the Revelator saw this kind of miracle working as part of the sixth angel of Revelation 16. In the language of his figurative speech he accurately described the holistic health movement as it joined the stream of Eastern religions and self-centered neopaganism.

> The sixth angel poured out his bowl on the great river Euphrates, and its water was dried up to prepare the way for the kings from the East. Then I saw three evil spirits that looked like frogs; they came out of the mouth of the dragon, out of the mouth of the beast and out of the mouth of the false prophet. They are spirits of demons performing miraculous signs, and they go out to the kings of the whole world, to gather them for the battle on the great day of God Almighty. Behold, I come like a thief![14]

Chapter Six

ACUPUNCTURE AND REFLEXOLOGY

According to Chinese tradition, it was discovered that warriors who received arrow wounds in certain anatomical locations developed anesthesia, or numbness, in other areas of their bodies. Over a 1500-year span of time, a written summary of the practice of acupuncture developed and was published under the name of "Nei Ching." The first of these thirty-four volumes was written 4,500 years ago. Thus, if we were to accept the date of these documents, they were being written in a period shortly after the world Flood and extending to the time of Moses. Famous and honored physicians in China were practicing the art of acupuncture concurrently with Christ who used the power of His Father to heal. Pien Chueh, a physician of this era, is said to have healed a patient in a coma by acupuncture. This healing was followed by twenty days of herbal therapy leading to complete health of the patient, a prince, whose funeral arrangements had to be canceled.

From the experience of the wounded warriors, the concept developed that the size of the wound did not influence the effectiveness of the penetration therapy or acupuncture. Therefore, it was possible to use stone instruments that were thinner and smaller in size than the arrows, a fact which must have contributed to the comfort of the patients. In time, the stone tools were replaced by wood or bamboo. Later, metal needles were used, making the therapy even more effective.

Even though acupuncture has had a long and illustrious history in China, there was a period from 1929–1958 when it was outlawed. At the urging of Chairman Mao's wife, it was brought back into political favor during the turmoil of the "Cultural Revolution." When the United States, then under President Nixon, re-established cultural ties with China, acupuncture was observed for the first time by modem Western scientists.

Acupuncture is thought to be effective by "unblocking" disturbances within an external energy system. This concept is completely unrelated to the anatomical system of nerves, veins, arteries, and lymphatics that has been carefully documented by scientists of all races and religions in medical centers all over the world. In distinction from anatomical understanding, the energy system of acupuncture is similar to the "aura" of the Hindu system as discussed in a previous chapter. "The theory behind acupuncture is that there exists in the body the dual flows of energy called 'Yin' and 'Yang' contained within an overall conception of energy known as the 'Chi' or 'life force'."[1] As with the chakra system, this energy is seen as part of an all-pervasive universal power which arose from the cosmic "someplace out there." Yang originated from the sun and stars and is visualized as dominant, good, positive, and male. An opposing force, Yin, originated from the earth and the moon and is represented as evil, negative, and female. According to this theorized system, the eternal quest for peace, health, and happiness for both the individual and the universe is the balance of these two opposing forces.

On the body's surface, this alleged energy force is organized into twenty-four channels or meridians that flow longitudinally from head to toe. These meridians correspond to internal organs of generally understood anatomy (i.e. lungs, stomach, heart, etc.). However, there are several rather strange entities such as "triple warmer" and "circulation" that do not fit any known anatomical part! This fact is conveniently left out of most modern discussions on the subject.

Along the meridians are points of "low resistance," which are the actual acupuncture sites. These are stimulated with blunt pressure, mechanical needle motion, electricity, and the burning of bits of leaf or herbal compound. Traditionally, there are over 800 acupuncture sites, but new ones are being "discovered" by modern therapists. The number of sites needed to produce anesthesia seems to be quite variable. A standard thoracotomy, that opens into the chest cavity through an incision six to eight inches long by the removal of a rib, has typically required eighteen sites. More recently, however, some clinics for surgery are now using only one. In some cases, no needles at all are used for complete anesthesia.[2] This extreme variation in technique certainly raises the question of subjectivism and is very unphysiological.

According to Chinese teaching, even the external ear represents the entire body in "microcosm" and can be used for diagnosis and treatment. The claim has been made that the meridian lines fit anatomical and physiological principles; however, there is no serious evidence that has been presented to document this hypothesis.

Despite these weaknesses and lack of rational physiological explanation, acupuncture does work in some cases. A certain percentage of those receiving this treatment will have sufficient anesthesia for a surgical operation. Those patients who are quite stoical and passive will be much more adaptable to this form of therapy than will those who are more independent and aggressive. For this reason, it is unlikely that anesthesia by acupuncture will ever become widely used in the Western world for surgical procedures, even though it may be accepted for "recreational medicine" or a form of social therapy.

Dr. John de Romanett in his book *Acupuncture, Mesmerism and Hypnotism,* makes a strong case for the relationship between acupuncture and hypnosis. His thesis is based on the concept of monotonous, repetitive stimuli through either manipulation of needles, electrical current, or sound. He points out that even animals can be hypnotized and anesthetized through these methods.[3] His observations are confirmed by Dr.

William Kraper and reported in the *Journal of the American Medical Association,* May 15, 1972.

It would seem strange that techniques with little or no physiological correlation, that have been developed from a spiritualistic culture, and are being practiced largely by those who believe and promote an anti-Christian philosophy, would attract Christians. But they do! And many are opening themselves to the fallacies of Eastern philosophies based on an attempt to balance opposites, such as good and evil, or male and female. Christianity, in contrast, is based on the Biblical truth of the triumph of good over evil.

Two Christian authors, who have made some very useful comments on the holistic health movement, have used strange words in offering acceptance to the practice of acupuncture.

> First, we propose that entry into the realm of ancient Chinese medicine be made for only one specific reason: the treatment of chronic pain with counter-stimulation therapy, such as needling or electrical stimulation, when other methods have failed or are only partially successful.... We feel it is important that the therapist be thinking in terms of mechanisms in the nervous system, rather than in terms of meridians and life energy.[4] *Thinking so doesn't make it right!*

Sad to say, this same line of reasoning is similar to that used by King Saul when he justified his visit to the witch of Endor. Saul had indeed "expelled the mediums and spiritists from the land."[5] But now Samuel was dead, and David had been anointed king apparent. "When Saul saw the Philistine army, he was afraid; terror filled his heart. He inquired of the Lord, but the Lord did not answer him by dreams or Urim or prophets. Saul then said to his attendants, 'Find me a woman who is a medium, so I may go and inquire of her.' "[6]

The seeming lack of alternatives is not a good reason to resort to methods that are clearly objectionable and that could lead to our eternal destruction. As harsh as it may sound, chronic pain may be preferable to giving ourselves over to a healer or a technique that is clearly anti-physiological, anti-logical, and anti-Christ.

It is important, however, to point out that there are true, physiological methods used by physical therapists and others that do stimulate nerves of the body and do block pain pathways. These practitioners make no attempt to "balance energies." Instead, stimulation of the regular nerves of the body can block pain sensation, and has been helpful in many chronic pain problems. An example of this method is the "Transcutaneous nerve stimulator." Counterirritation with massage would also illustrate the same method. As is often the case, the false lies very close to the true.

Reflexology is a close cousin to acupuncture. Even though seen as a more acceptable "Western variety" of the energy-balancing technique, its roots are deeply planted in the soil of spiritism. In fact, the same meridian lines of acupuncture apply to reflexology. The technique is based on the idea that upon the surface of the palm of the hand and the sole of the foot are energy centers correlating with the organs of the body. The big toe is of considerable importance in the practice of reflexology. In mystical Zoroastrian tradition, the great toe is also important as a connection to the mind and can bring harmony to the body. Again, the idea of "energy congestion" or imbalance is reported to be the cause of disease. The massage of the foot or hand, according to the reflexologist, will locate little "crystals" of "congested energy." This congested area is usually tender to touch and with proper massage will disappear. Despite the microscopic evaluation of the skin and nervous system of the hand and foot, these points of energy congestion have never been demonstrated by those who have made careful study of the human anatomy. If the reflexology therapist is feeling something that is not there and manipulating energy that cannot be demonstrated, what is the reason for his success? "Success" does come, and at times the diagnosis is accurate. Is there a mediumistic quality to this apparently effective technique which is similar to the reading of the aura or use of the divining rod? This is a difficult question for us to ask, for many "good" Christian people are involved in reflexology both as therapists and as patients. In evaluating this, it is important to set aside feelings, pride, and prejudice, and carefully evaluate not only the immediate results, but also the eternal consequences. The Holy Spirit directs most clearly by the Inspired Word, not by some rather vague impression which can be strongly influenced by personal feelings and experiences. The Christian should be able to easily identify this technique as being dangerous because of its association with "energy balancing," for the Scriptures plainly tell us to avoid "divination."[7]

Chapter Seven

APPLIED AND BEHAVIORAL KINESIOLOGY

Kinesiology is simply the study of the function, structure, and action of muscles. In the last few decades, much has been learned in physiology laboratories that has formed the basis of our understanding of exercise and calisthenics. In the physical rehabilitation of those suffering from paralysis, the information available regarding the action of muscle groups has been very helpful. The Christian can relate well to this type of study, as it demonstrates the wonders of the body that God has made.

In distinction to the true science of kinesiology, applied and behavioral kinesiology have very little to do with the legitimate physiological study of muscles.

In 1963 George Goodheart, a chiropractor, combined his study of "acupuncture, massage, acupressure, the very dangerous occult system of Kundalini yoga, and polarity therapy" to reinvent applied kinesiology.[1]

The basic theory revolves around the "Chi" life force, and therefore is closely associated with the theory of acupuncture and the aura. Applied kinesiology is used as a diagnostic tool to locate "imbalances" in energy fields. By this method, it is claimed that nutritional, environmental, or even psychological imbalances and deficiencies can be determined. When supplementation of specific nutrients is undertaken, the precise amount needed is said to be determined by using muscle weakness or strength as the indicator. Although the average practitioner of applied kinesiology may use only simple resistive testing of muscle groups, some rather sophisticated equipment such as the Cybex Dynamometer or the Bio—My kinesiometer can also be used to record electronically the amount of energy expended by a muscle group. The dials, switches, and "gizmos" give the techniques a semblance of respectability, and an air of scientific credibility.

The following quotation from *A Visual Encyclopedia of Unconventional Medicine* will help to illustrate the strange collection of fact and fancy that forms the basis of this therapy. Beneath a picture of a patient lying on his back with the therapist exerting downward pressure on his uplifted leg, the following comment is made.

> In this picture, the 'fascia lata' is being tested. This is the muscle which helps to flex or bend the thigh, to draw it away from the body sideways, and keep it turned in. The patient lies face upward with the leg raised to 45 degrees and slightly to the side. The therapist exerts pressure against the outside of the leg to push the leg down and in. If the muscle is weak, this indicates intestinal problems of constipation, spastic colon, colitis or diarrhea. It can be remedied by nutritional supplementation.[2]

The "fascia lata" is a dense fibrous sheet which covers the tensor fascia lata muscle. The various gastrointestinal problems mentioned have various causes and could not be diagnosed by weakness in a specific muscle, and considerably less by its fibrous covering. Whether these symptoms, which may represent anything from colon cancer to a viral gastroenteritis, could be relieved by "nutritional supplementation" is highly questionable.

John Diamond, M.D., added another whimsical concept to applied kinesiology and called it behavioral kinesiology (BK). Perhaps more from his study of the meaning of the word "thymus" or from his Eastern mystical leanings rather than from any real understanding of body physiology, he conceived the idea that the thymus gland is the "master gland" and controls the energy of the meridians. In his book, *Your Body Doesn't Lie,* Dr. Diamond gives a rehearsal of the origin of the Greek word "thymos," which is the root word for "thymus." Galen, an anatomist of the second century, chose the word thymus to describe the small pinkish-gray organ located in the anterior chest cavity. Galen had no understanding of the function of this organ at that time. He was influenced, however, by the prevailing meaning of "thymos" as consciousness or the spirit.

Dr. Diamond refers to Julian Jaynes as the authority on "thymos." In the *Iliad,* by Homer, says Jaynes, the gods "told" men what to do and how to feel. In this first "objective" phase in the development of Greek consciousness, thymos meant motion or activity as externally perceived. But later, the gods' voices faded away, or displayed a fallibility that dismayed the mortals—and "thymos" became internalized (the second phase) and took on a more active role. Keyed up for battle, man strained to hear the commands of yore. From his stress came physical changes—a rise in adrenaline, a quickening of the heartbeat, and a corresponding "fluttering in the breast." In time, these internal responses to stress became associated with "thymos" itself. In the subjective phase of the evolution of consciousness, "thymos" was regarded as a "container" into which strength could be put. It was also personified. "Thymos" talked to man (and man to "thymos"); it gave him strength for warring and urged him on to love and victory. Thus conversant with man, "thymos" came to be compared to man, and was given qualities that lifted it from the realm of things to that of persons.[3]

Tracing the evolution of Homer's "consciousness" outlines the basis and origins of monastic and humanistic thought and theology. Man first becomes dissatisfied with the "God out there." This dissatisfaction led to the idea that "I am my god." God then became mankind, and humanism was the source of reference and strength.

Except for this philosophical departure in the appendix of his book, Dr. Diamond generally presents behavioral kinesiology in physiological terms. Since we have developed a certain amount of awe for the medical profession, these ideas, expressed by a medical doctor, can easily lead people into the practice of behavioral kinesiology.

I believe it is of considerable significance that this pseudoscientific explanation of the relationship of the thymus gland to "energy" is closely akin to the "chakra" theory as discussed in Chapter Four. Note carefully the similarity of thinking between the two statements as quoted below.

> A major discovery of behavioral kinesiology is that the thymus gland monitors and regulates energy flow in the meridian system.... The controller of energy flow in the body is the thymus gland. Day after day, moment by moment, it monitors and re-balances our Life Energy.[4]

> The throat chakra, which focuses sixteen petals of light, is the power center in man.... The shortening of the days, or the cycles, of the balancing of karma occurs through the correct use of the spoken word.... Anything and everything that proceeds from the throat chakra coalesces in form, for good or for ill, by the action of the power of the word.[5]

The similarity of thought, even though one is couched in very metaphysical terms and the other in somewhat scientific wording, is no accident, as both have a common root in mystical religions.

I once knew an avowed psychic and Satanist who operated a health food store and practiced behavioral kinesiology. When a group of Christians became interested in this form of healing, he was quite amused with their dabbling in the occult arts as he recognized and practiced them. He was able to demonstrate that he could make a person weak or strong by just thinking "thoughts" of love or hate as he went through the standard muscle testing technique of behavioral kinesiology. I marvel that with such clear connections with spiritism, behavioral kinesiology would be practiced by sincere Christians. My psychic friend used most of the holistic health techniques. He had a right to feel comfortable in their use, since he worked closely with the power that originated them.

Chapter Eight

IRIDOLOGY

The eye has fascinated both philosopher and physician alike. For centuries this "seat of the soul" has been analyzed and studied with fascination. Even David commented on the condition of his eyes while suffering under the guilt of his sin with Bathsheba, saying, "even the light has gone from my eyes."[1] The eye contact is a point of communication and a point of personal identity. Medicine has always given considerable emphasis to the eye during physical examination. Signs of liver failure can be detected by the sclera, or white of the eye, turning yellow. Hypertension and diabetes are often diagnosed by viewing the retina and its complex structures.

> Herpes zoster has been associated with a severe iritis, eventually ending in a hyperpigmentation and necrosis of the iris. In neurofibromatosis (von Recklinghausen's disease), one may find, among other ocular manifestations, areas of pigmentation that are sometimes incorrectly diagnosed as melanosis. Tuberculosis, diabetes mellitus, atherosclerosis, sarcoidosis, and rheumatic disorders (Reiter's syndrome, ulcerative colitis, Crohn's disease, juvenile rheumatoid arthritis, and ankylosing spondylitis) are among a few of the disorders and syndromes too numerous to mention with confirmed manifestations in the iris.[2]

This medical quotation documents the fact that the iris of the eye can become affected by many disease processes that will color or cause breakdown of the structures of the eye. Ignoring these physiological mechanisms, the iridologist divides the iris into ninety-six zones and multiple minor areas that are related to various anatomical parts of the body. A diagnosis is then made by noting the pigmentation of these zones. Blue is healthy, but grey or brown imply disease. Even though most diagnostic work is done with a hand lens, there is rather sophisticated photographic equipment that is used for permanent documentation. According to Jessica Maxwell, who wrote the book *The Eye-Body Connection*, the "basis for iridology is the neuro-optic reflex, an intimate marriage of the estimated half million nerve filaments of the iris with the cervical ganglia of the sympathetic nervous system. The neuro-optic reflex turns the iris into an organic etch-a-sketch that monitors impressions from all over the body as they come in."[3]

The iris of the eye is connected to the sympathetic nervous system, but it is hardly the nerve center for the whole body, nor is it a permanent record of life events. A very interesting study has already been reported in the *Journal of the American Medical Association* in 1979. Dr. Allie Simon and others made an honest attempt to evaluate the accuracy of iridology. To avoid the factors of personal contact, only photographs of the eye were used for evaluation. The kidney zone was chosen because this is a prominent zone in iridology, and kidney function can be easily assessed with creatinine blood tests. Three prominent iridologists agreed to participate. From photographs of the iris, they were to determine which of the patients had laboratory confirmed kidney failure and which were normal. Three ophthalmologists were also shown the photographs and their results were recorded.

The diagnostic accuracy of five observers was less than random chance. The sixth observer, an experienced iridologist, was able to achieve an accuracy of 95% in selecting those patients with severe renal failure. His ability to diagnose the presence of kidney disease approached the accuracy of a blood test. Yet, in the process, he diagnosed 88% of those with normal renal function as having kidney failure. Thus, his apparent accuracy occurred by making the diagnosis of kidney failure in almost all of the tested patients. This testing led to the conclusion that iridology has the double jeopardy of giving a false diagnosis of renal disease to many normal individuals. When taken as a whole, iridology missed an accurate diagnosis in 75% of those that did have significant disease.

There is reason for concern regarding the inaccuracy of this diagnostic method. Yet, at times it is very accurate, to which many patients can attest. If there is no scientifically valid reason for the ability of the iridologist to diagnose disease, is it possible that there is a psychic quality to this methodology?

The metaphysical bend of those who practice iridology is apparent in comments such as those by Dr. Carter.

> Intuitive skills do come into play here, and whether we want to call this "psychic" ability or not (it remains to be defined.... What do we mean by 'psychic'? Is that just a paranormal state? It is very easy to label it as such. We may find that these skills are just a further progression of the conscious ability of an individual.... a kind of hyperconscious or ultraconscious state.[4]

Kurt Koch, in his book *The Devil's Alphabet,* is a bit more blunt in his evaluation.

> Many of our healers and occult practitioners use eye-diagnosis mediumistically rather than medically. That means that they are only interested in the iris as a mediumistic contact. In this way the human eye serves a psychometric purpose in much the same way as hand lines do when a fortune-teller uses them as contact material or as an 'intuition stimulant.' When this is the case, eye-diagnosis becomes a form of fortune-telling. Because of this, these eye-diagnosticians are often very successful. Indeed some of them with little or no medical training can diagnose illness with 100% accuracy.[5]

Iridology definitely has occult roots. "Stone slabs have been found in Asia Minor depicting the iris and its relationship to the rest of the body. The Chaldeans of Babylon, who carved the slabs, were known as soothsayers."[6] We may think the originators of iridology were men like Ignatz von Peczely, who published his findings in 1881 or Pastor Felks who lived during the same period of time, but in reality, this system of divination is very ancient.

It is more than mere coincidence that the eye chart zones are divided into ninety-six compartments. This is exactly the number of divisions in the "third-eye chakra" of the aura and the occultic external energy system based firmly in Hinduism.

> We return to the absolute consciousness of God through the third-eye chakra, which has ninety-six petals. The third eye, vibrating in the emerald green of the science of truth, gives us the immaculate picture of individuals, of civilizations, of the divine pattern.... The third-eye always gives you the immaculate concept of the blueprint of life as well as the discrimination to know good and evil.[7]

These ninety-six petals of the third-eye chakra give the "blueprint of life" just as the ninety-six zones of iridology give the "diagnosis of life." The similarity is too obvious to overlook.

The mediumistic quality or supernatural ability of iridology is very similar to what occurred in the practice of phrenology. With this method, diagnosis was made from the irregular configuration of the skull of an individual instead of the iris. Robert Collyer, M.D., wrote the book, *Psychography, or the Embodiment of Thought: with an Analysis of Phreno-Magnetism, Neurology and Mental Hallucination, Including Rules to Govern and Produce the Magnetic State,* in which he records the signed testimony of one of his patients.

> I now declare that Dr. Robert H. Collyer has acted on the various portions of my head as located by the phrenologists to correspond with certain faculties of the mind. When the part was acted on the function of which I was acquainted with, the result followed; that is, if I knew Dr. C. was acting on the organ of Combativeness, I felt quarrelsome; or if the organ of Mirthfulness, I could not help laughing, etc. But when I did not know the function of the part acted on, no result followed. This proves to my mind that the effect pro-

duced when I was conscious of the function of the part to be acted upon, was produced by striking my mind so as to produce a result independent of my will....[8]

Phrenology became a prominent medical practice in the 1800's. "In fact, phrenology almost became a religion. Queen Victoria had her children's heads read by a phrenologist, and Karl Marx was a firm believer in the 'science.' "[9] This type of divination of the state of health by surface, non-physiological exam was clearly warned against at that time.

"The sciences of phrenology, psychology, and mesmerism are the channel through which he [Satan] comes more directly to this generation and works with that power which is to characterize his efforts near the close of probation."[10] I believe we are seeing that same power working today and well-meaning Christians are accepting it because "the coming of the lawless one will be in accordance with the work of Satan displayed in all kinds of counterfeit miracles, signs and wonders, and in every sort of evil that deceives those who are perishing. They perish because they refused to love the truth and so be saved."[11]

God has called us in this end-time to separate from everything of the occult and from Babylon. The call is to "Come out of her, my people, so that you will not share in her sins."[12] This is not a time to see how close we can get to these practices, but a time to be completely separate. Separate now!

Chapter Nine

HERBAL THERAPY

Then the angel showed me the river of the water of life, as
clear as crystal flowing from the throne of God and of the
Lamb down the middle of the great street of the city.... And
the leaves of the trees were for the healing of the nations.[1]

As John the Revelator viewed this majestic scene of the
Heavenly city, he put into words the eternal hope that vegetable
matter would and could heal the ills of mankind. Even though
this was "heavenly vegetable matter" and the source of its
effectiveness was God's own power, he could describe what
he saw only in terms that he and his society understood at that
point in history.

The annals of medical care are replete with the concept of
herbal therapy. From antiquity, stories come to us of the triumph of these therapies. Even in ancient prose, Virgil, a wild
goat, is depicted as being healed from a wound caused by an
archer's arrow, when the goat instinctively sought out the herb
dittany (*Origanum dictatamnam*).[2]

The Ebers Papyrus, dated 1500 B.C., details scores of herbs
used for medicinal purposes. It is possible that Moses may have
been taught these therapies while he was being trained in Egypt
for leadership as a ruler, priest, and physician. John Parkinson,
the great English herbalist, documented 3,800 medicinal plants
in his exhaustive work *Theatrum Botanicum* written in 1640.
From this common herbal background sprang two main lines
of medical reasoning. Allopathy emerged using herbal agents
which have an action different from, or contrary to, the symptom of the disease being treated. As an example, willow bark

46

tea is given to lower an elevated body temperature. The dosage is increased until the desired effect is achieved.

Homeopathy took the opposite direction. An herbal agent would be chosen that gave the same effect as the symptom to be treated. If a person was nauseated, an agent that caused nausea would be prescribed. The dosage would be decreased by diluting the agent repeatedly, thus giving less and less of the agent until only the "energy" remained.

Even though allopathy, or regular Western medical practice as carried out today, takes the "drugging business" beyond its rightful bounds and often fails to educate the patient in areas of health preservation, it at least follows the natural laws of physiology rather than the mystical "energy" concepts of homeopathy. The facts of body mechanics have not been developed by practitioners attempting to prove their bias or sell a product. Instead, scientists have studied the body function for pure knowledge. These results have been retested by other researchers and confirmed in different laboratories. This information can be used by the conscientious medical practitioner to develop a beneficial therapy or a preventive plan. Herbs have formed the basis for many of the pharmaceutical preparations. Digitalis, aspirin, and some pain relievers have their origin in herbology. Major drug companies have teams of scientists who evaluate tribal and folklore treatments, looking for useful therapies. All plant substances are complex groups of chemical agents. Instead of being "simple," as is often heralded by health food enthusiasts, they are much more complex than a single pharmaceutical preparation.

> ...The dried leaf of Digitalis purpurea L. has long been used in the treatment of congestive heart failure. It contains approximately thirty different glycosides which possess some cardiotonic properties.[3]

Each glycoside has its own separate effect, time of onset, and duration of action. Herbalists often claim that the action of the whole leaf or root is greater than the combined effect of the components taken separately. This claim violates all physical laws and smacks of a supernatural mysticism or "energy enhancement."

Yet herbs are useful in the treatment of disease. This fact has been confirmed by generations of people who have used the medicinal herbs effectively. Diligent effort must be put forth to discover which herbal "drugs" can give the most benefit and the fewest side effects to man.

Within this context, there are times when herbs or "botanical therapies" may be valuable allies to good lifestyle practices. The more healthful our way of life, the less frequently will we need the acute intervention of herbal drugs and therapies. When botanical drugs are used, it would be wise to understand the chemistry and pharmacology of that which is used. Sadly, much of the herbal information is either outdated or has never been tested. Worse yet, some of it has been taken from occult sources. The "herbal astrologist," Nicholas Culpepper, has been enthusiastically accepted by the children of the "Age of Aquarius" or "New Age." The reason for this acceptance is obvious. His use of astrological explanations for the effect of herbs fits well with "New Age" thinking. Along with the occult influence has also come physically dangerous information. According to Culpepper's reasoning, "Lily-of-the-valley" (*Convallaria majalis L.*) is not poisonous. Yet research has indicated that it contains the most toxic cardiac glycoside in existence.

Many of the American Indian herbal mixtures have been formulated during states of trance with the "Great Spirit." Other mixtures are based on a mystical Chinese system of balancing Yin and Yang "energies." The American, Elizabeth Bellhouse, claimed to have been led by a "spirit guide" to develop a therapy she called "Vita Florum." Through the use of her "intuitive mind," she was instructed to pick certain species of herbs and flowers and combine them for treatment purposes. The plants were then to be held over water and exposed to sunlight in order to transfer a "healing radiation" to the water. This therapy, she claimed, "heals the body because it is a harmonizing agent that opens the way for psychological and Spiritual growth."[4]

Bach "flower remedies" were developed by Dr. Bach in the early nineteen hundreds. He was strongly influenced by Dr. Hahnemann, the founder of homeopathy, and gave up his orthodox practice of medicine for homeopathic treatments. By his own admission, he next gave up the search for scientific validation of the therapies he was using and began to use his "intuitive faculty." Using this method, he then found that he could experience the action of the flowering herbs by just holding his hand near it. The flower thus chosen was then placed in water and exposed to the sunlight for three hours or gently boiled in water. This extract was then used most often for emotional states such as panic, fear, loneliness, depression, and lack of confidence. Who needs God if "flower water" will do the same thing? One of the remedies developed would even help overcome the "overcare" for the welfare of others.

Two principles can be made clear about herbs. First, herbs can be effective in cases of sickness, but should not be used as an everyday potion. God abundantly supplied, in the fruits, grains, nuts and vegetables, that which is necessary for maintenance of vibrant health on a day-by-day basis. Second, single agents should be prescribed, not multiple mixtures of dubious origins.

One nineteenth-century Christian author wrote,

> There are many simple herbs which, if our nurses would learn the value of, they could use in the place of drugs, and find effective. Many times I have been applied to for advice as to what should be done in cases of sickness or accident, and I have mentioned some of these simple remedies, and they have proved helpful.[5]

> The Lord has given some simple herbs of the field that at times are beneficial; and if every family were educated in how to use these herbs in case of sickness, much suffering might be prevented, and no doctor need be called. These old fashioned, simple herbs, used intelligently, would have re-

covered many sick who would have died under drug medication.[6]

God's servants should not administer medicines which they know will leave behind injurious effects upon the system, even if they do relieve present suffering. Every poisonous preparation in the vegetable and mineral kingdoms, taken into the system, will leave its wretched influence, affecting the liver and lungs, and deranging the system generally.[7]

"Poisonous preparations" certainly are not solely produced in pharmaceutical factories. Wormwood contains a toxic substance called thujone. It causes convulsions in rats, and affects the human brain at the same site and in a similar way as marijuana. Wormwood was an ingredient in some alcoholic beverages until outlawed by various European countries. It was while under the influence of one of these beverages that the painter Vincent van Gogh cut off his own ear and sent it to a lady friend. Pokeroot, which has been recommended for almost every one of man's ills, contains a very toxic saponin mixture called phytolaccatoxin. "Children have died and adults have been hospitalized from the gastroenteritis, hypotension, and diminished respiration caused by eating pokeroot or the berries or leaves of the plant."[8] The principal agent in Chaparral or greasewood is nordihydroguaiaretic acid (NDGA), a potent antioxidant, which was thought to have anti-cancer properties. It, too, is quite toxic and will produce lesions in the mesenteric lymph nodes and kidneys of experimental animals.

Herbs for therapy? Certainly, but with the same caution we would use with any other substance or drug taken into the body.

Chapter Ten

THE ROOTS OF HEALING METHODS

Homeopathy

Samuel Christian Hahnemann stated in his original paper, published in 1796, that the basic tenant of homeopathy is *"similia, similibus curantur,"* or "like heals like." If a person was vomiting, homeopathy would recommend an herb or other chemical substance that caused vomiting. Dr. Hahnemann was led to this belief by observing that peruvian bark, a crude form of quinine, when given to a normal person, would produce a fever similar to that caused by malaria. When peruvian bark was given to a patient with malarial fever, Dr. Hahneman observed that the patient improved. From this experience, he concluded and assumed that this method would work in all diseases. Sadly, neither the action of quinine nor the pathology of malaria was understood at that time. This erroneous reasoning, based on inadequate information and a mystical mind-set, led Dr. Hahnemann to believe that disease was not caused by physical agents, but by "spirits."

> The natural disease is never to be considered as a noxious material situated somewhere within the interior or exterior of man but as one produced by an inimical spirit-like agency which, like a kind of infection disturbs in its instinctive existence of the spirit-like (conceptual) principle of life within the organism, torturing it as an evil spirit, and compelling it to produce certain ailments and disorders in the regular course of its life.[1]

This mystical view of the body's mechanics and health was in support of the animal magnetism movement of Anton Mesmer. Homeopathy's most astonishing feature is that the effectiveness of a potion is inversely proportional to the quantity of the active ingredient. This is like saying that the less salt used in the food, the saltier it tastes. Most cooks would consider this idea profoundly ridiculous. This seeming contradiction to "the way things are" is explained by Dr. Hahnemann with another mystical principle called "succussion." In this procedure, an agent is mixed in a particular way that causes "energy" to be transferred to the solution. These principles are followed in homeopathic laboratories in America and Europe today. A fresh sample of material, either animal, plant, or mineral in origin, is extracted with alcohol. This is called the "mother tincture." Sixty milligrams of the extract are then added to ten parts of alcohol, water, or sugar, and the mixture is then "succussed." From this dilution then, one part is diluted in ten parts to form the next dilution. As this dilution process is continued, the potency is increased up to one hundred thousand.

> In the case of one widely used remedy, 'Natrum Muriaticum,' or common salt, a single molecule weighs ten to the minus twenty-fourth power in milligrams. It follows that at a potency of thirty, not a single molecule of the original salt is likely to remain in the dose. Hahnemann's discovery, therefore, was that the power of a substance is not in the material but in its pattern. The further removed the material becomes, the greater the power of the pattern.[2]

It is difficult to find an appropriate comment to this quotation. First, ordinary table salt is the agent which is diluted to the point that not one molecule of salt is left. If this dilution is now "nothing" except water, what is doing the healing? From where is this "power" coming? These questions have concerned several Christian authors who quote homeopathists themselves for the answer.

The concept of the 'life force' is predominant in both holistic health and homeopathy. Margutti relates homeopathy to Burr's L-fields (for life). Dr. Gray refers to generalized life force that does the healing and states it has many names— chi, prana, spirit, etc. He gives the force almost a god-like power, providing, of course, it is stimulated by homeopathy…. Also of concern is the emphasis in homeopathy upon matching treatment to personalities, not disease, and here we come into a more clearly discernible possibility for occultism. Michaud states: "In homeopathy, we try to do that ®, which is why we have to put more stress on individual differences, and that leads to an interest in such things as astrology and acupuncture."[3]

Homeopathy, as practiced today, often disregards the importance of seeking the disease origin or emphasizing preventive or lifestyle factors in the maintenance of health. This failing is certainly not unique to homeopathy, since standard medical care often does the same. It is so easy to give a potion or pill and not worry about the need for a lifestyle change. This shift of emphasis was noted at a health institution that was functioning in the 1800's. "When Dr. A came to the Health Retreat, she laid aside her knowledge and practice of hygiene, and administered the little homeopathic doses for almost every ailment. This was against the light God had given."[4]

Homeopathy is given credit for curing everything from cancer to allergies. "By 'cure' the homeopath means relief from the ailment for life after being given one dose of one remedy (or at least only a very few remedies), and without being dependent on any regimen of activity, diet, or medication."[5]

Many fine Christian people practice homeopathy, but it is a delusion. The origin and association with the occultic practices cause us to recommend that we not "walk where angels fear to tread."

Chiropractic

Another practitioner that was deeply influenced by Anton Mesmer and animal magnetism was D.D. Palmer, the founder of chiropractic therapy. A magnetic healer in his own right, Palmer was an associate of Phineas Quimby, who developed the "New Thought Movement" of the mid-19th century. (Quimby also "healed" Mary Baker Eddy who started the Christian Science cult.) It was this mystical association that led Palmer to develop the concept that "life force" communicated through the nerves of the spinal cord which exited from the vertebral column. A misalignment of the spine would therefore block the flow of "vital force" according to the theory. It is true that nerves with electrical potentials do indeed exit from the spine, but certainly not a "life force" or "spirit."

The chiropractor of today places much emphasis on the proper adjustment of the spinal column. To the casual observer and to many chiropractors, the practice begins and ends with manipulation and body mechanics. However, the roots of this "art" are firmly planted in the occult. The son of D.D. Palmer was the energetic B.J. Palmer, who did the most to develop his father's observations into a system of health. He was able to articulate the function of the "innate," a mystical spirit guide.

> While trying to find my way out of these dilemmas, I took a new look at the basic chiropractic concept of 'innate.' This philosophy insisted that the primal source of energy or vital force (innate) is directed through the nervous system,…innate was that power which kept the complicated autonomic system functioning. Innate was Infinite Life expressing itself through an individual for a specific period in time and space.[6]

The "innate" of the patient can communicate with the "innate" of the practitioner, and greater healing is said to occur. Some chiropractors speak of letting their minds flow with the innate which helps them know where to massage or manipulate. It is the innate that causes Christians great concern. B.J. Palmer attributed his accomplishments to his innate or the "inner fellow." In fact, when speaking about his accomplishments, he always used the pronoun "we." "I have achieved nothing. I do nothing. It is innate that does the work."[7]

We must be very careful not to label all chiropractic therapy as occult. However, since there is the potential of occultic training and therapy in the chiropractic field, it would be wise to know the philosophy of your "healer."

Western Medicine

To be certain, Western medicine also has origins that will make one's hair stand on end. The caduceus, or symbol of medicine, is an everyday reminder that Western medicine is also deeply grounded in the occult. "Thoth, Hermes, and Mercury gods of Egypt, Greece, and Rome are identical to Cush, son of Ham. Cush, an early Mesopotamian leader, introduced the basic ideas for magic, which was later recognized as a part of the Babylonian mysteries."[8] Alchemists were the original physicians. They attempted to blend base metals into gold, black into white, and good with evil. Even their stills were shaped like an intertwining serpent. The "single snake" caduceus can be traced to the god Asclepius, who has somewhat better credentials than the other gods. "The Apocalypse condemns sorcery which included those associated with alchemy, magic, and witchcraft. The Greek word for sorcery, *pharmakeia*, is a term from which we have derived the English word pharmacy."[9] While we cannot condemn all medications, it is interesting that the drugs of today are a blending of "good" and "evil." Even a cursory look through the *Physician's Desk Reference* will demonstrate that the expected value of a drug must be weighed against its harmful side effects. In contrast, the preventive lifestyle approach to medical care that God has ordained has no side effects. It produces only good and salubrious benefits to body, mind, and spirit. Fortunately for us today, certain German physicians turned away from mystical medicine during the late nineteenth century and developed the "rational school" of medical thinking. Anatomy, physiology, pathology, and chemistry became the basis for Western medicine. While it has become quite mechanistic, and certainly far from "holistic," it has, to a fault, attempted to be free from "spirit." It is this lack of concern for the spiritual and social aspects of life that has driven many to seek alternative therapies. Despite this weakness, Western medicine and its preoccupation with the objective facts of life have made it possible to study the function of the body with candor and to be less influenced by mystical reference points.

As we can quickly see, there is no perfect therapy. For this reason, we must carefully seek forms of therapy that honor God and do not harm His handiwork.

> There are many ways of practicing the healing art, but there is only one way that Heaven approves. God's remedies are simple agencies of nature that will not tax or debilitate the system through their powerful properties. Pure air and water, cleanliness, a proper diet, purity of life, and a firm trust in God, are remedies for the want of which thousands are dying, yet these remedies are going out of date because their skillful use requires work that the people do not appreciate.[10]

Chapter Eleven

SELF-HELP

Janice is a thirty-five year old, midlevel corporation executive. She is married and has two children, ages 10 and 14. The children are bright achievers. Her husband is a busy attorney. Janice has headaches, bad headaches. The pain is so intense at times that she has actually considered suicide. The kids are on the move and demanding of her time and energy. Her husband is midlife and has little time for home or Janice. She must hold her own professionally now or bow out of the swift competition for advancement in her corporation. The headaches have been going on for two years. Somehow she has found time to see almost every medical specialist in town. The X-rays, CAT scans of the brain, and electrical muscle conduction tests have all been negative. There have been many referrals by frustrated physicians, who don't have the answer. Everyone just shrugs and says, "Your tests are all normal, Janice." But the pain...The pain goes on. No one stops to talk about the pain or the person who is about ready to collapse from the pain. "Who cares about the tests?" she thinks. "Doesn't anybody care about me?"

Janice is not a churchgoer, but she does have a few friends that are. They say that they are praying for her, but she is not sure what that means. She does know that whatever it is, it isn't working for her. She has even tried a few "prayers" herself. They seemed silly, almost like talking to herself.

One day at work, the corporation brought in a "Human Potential" expert to speak to the management staff. He discussed, in some detail, the relationship between thought processes and productivity. It was different from the "try harder" routine that she had so often heard before. The message that she was hearing now was more how to relax and "let the inner self go." "Self-realization" was the goal to achieve, because inside of you there is the potential of power and success if it is allowed to mature. It sounded so easy and certainly "good news" for the woman who had always "tried harder" at everything from homemaking to increasing corporate profits.

A few weeks later, she met a lovely woman from one of the other offices who invited her to a seminar on "Miracles." René seemed to have it all together, so to speak. There was a warmth and confidence that Janice admired. As far as the topic of discussion was concerned, she could certainly use a "miracle." The seminar took her by surprise. It was in a home, not in some cold, formal meeting room. The fellowship and warmth of the group was something that her starved spiritual nature quickly warmed to. They called themselves the "Caring People." The open attitude and hopefulness of everyone seemed almost like a religion to her, even though there were people of all religious persuasions there. She heard of others whose illnesses had disappeared as they achieved certain levels of awareness.

Since nothing else seemed to be working for her, she launched into this new experience with her usual gusto. Meeting once a week for these encounters, she learned about the "oneness of life." "We are part of the great whole," she was taught. "Nothing is ever lost." It did give her a feeling of belonging and seemed to answer the nagging question of what happens when one dies. She began to read some of Kubler-Ross's books on death and dying. The mystical "out of the body" experiences were especially fascinating to her, as she had been raised in a severely mechanical environment with little thought of spiritual things.

There was plenty of reading to do. She particularly liked the idea that there are many pathways that lead to truth. Here is an example of what her mind was feeding on.

> There are many paths up the mountain to enlightenment. But, when the paths get to the top, they all come together in

realization that truth is one. That is, when the 'ego dies and we are reborn into life, into reality.' In the enlightened condition, you discover that you are not just the traveler, you are also the path and the mountain.[1]

A new sense of power began to come into her life. And to think that she was doing all this through the power of her own mind, in connection with "Cosmic Consciousness." She felt as if life was just beginning.

> About the most critical point to be understood is this: the value of mystical and transformative states is not in producing some new experience, but in getting rid of the experiences. Getting rid, that is, of the egocentric consciousness which experiences life from a contracted, self-centered point of view rather than the free, unbound perspective of a sage who knows he or she is infinity operating through a finite form.[2]

The headaches were going away! Where modern technical medicine had failed, her newfound belief system had succeeded in a "miracle." There was, however, one area in her life that would not change. She could not stop smoking. Her husband said she lacked willpower, but she knew better than that. How could she now be frustrated in her search for complete health and inner enlightenment?

One day she received a brochure in the mail describing a stop-smoking program at a nearby Christian church. Why not? It would not hurt to try. The first evening at the church, she found a personal warmth of human contact similar to that which she had experienced at the "Miracle" seminar. Later, in the evening program, she was taken through a relaxation sequence of mind therapy. She had done this many times before when wanting to create a state of higher understanding and felt very familiar with the technique. She could tell who the experienced ones were and who were not. Some had a little trouble relaxing and "letting go." But they soon learned to respond to the soft light, and the deep, melodious voice of their leader.

Each participant received much affirmation that he or she would indeed stop smoking by just following this extremely successful program.

The second meeting included a film on the power of positive thought patterns. This certainly seemed compatible with the training received at work and at the "Miracle" seminars. The primary statement of the film was that you could do exactly what you set your mind to do. After the motion picture, a graying older gentleman introduced an optional component of the program. Most participants stayed for this part, which covered the area of "spiritual strength." Prayer was referred to as a technique or method of meditation. Ritualistically, you would ask fervently, believe as hard as you could, and claim or affirm that it had happened. Visualizing the power of God was said to help also. She could relate to this, but was a bit confused as to why it was optional or why it was needed, if the concepts portrayed in the film were adequate. At any rate, she had learned to accept all others in their pathway toward truth. Perhaps Christians needed a little extra help.

For better or worse, she did stop smoking. She was very pleased with herself for having overcome another hurdle in her life. It felt good to be in control and know that her mind could do almost anything. Through this experience she felt that her newfound Christian friends had helped her to another state of enlightenment.

About a week after she had finished the stop-smoking program, a young couple from the church stopped by to see how she was doing. It was a pleasure to be with these people again. During the conversation, they asked her if she would like to study about Jesus Christ. Now, Janice already knew about Jesus Christ. He was one of the ascended Fathers, who had used the method of enlightenment to live a life that was an example for all of us. This she had learned from the "Miracles" seminar. So it was with some awe and curiosity that she approached the subject as the young couple read about Jesus who "died for us." Martyrdom did seem to be the ultimate of "nothingness" and she was impressed. In their enthusiasm, the young people mistook her openness for a willingness to "be saved." She was assured that all she had to do was admit that she was a "sinner," ask for "forgiveness" and "believe." These terms were completely foreign to her. She had just stopped smoking, and now they wanted her to admit to being a "sinner," in need of "salvation." She had recently gotten over her headaches through becoming attuned to the "unity of the universe." She had become the "I am." Her performance at work had improved markedly. She was a better and more accepting mother and wife. And now these people wanted to give her "salvation." It all sounded a bit strange. She had learned at the Christian smoking cessation program that even the hardest and most difficult habits can be overcome with the use of the human will. Regaining her composure and assuming the forgiveness attitude that she had learned at the "Miracle" seminar, she quietly showed the Christians to the door. She did not need any of their "negative vibrations" with this "sin" business.

This scenario is just a sample of the inroads being made into our culture by numerous self-help philosophies and encounter groups. From the workplace to the media and entertainment fields, it is ever present. Sadly, even the Christian church has followed the "Eastern way" by trying to secularize and make its programs more "human" and germane to the society of today.

The reason we as Christians are so vulnerable to the self-help movement, and even bring it into our teaching and outreach, is that we have forgotten why Christ came to this earth in the first place. Our center of understanding goes no further than ourselves. God is seen as a magician that is just waiting for me to ask for another trick. We may want to be beautiful, wealthy, and smart, but His will for our lives may be quite different from our wants.

Calvin Miller has written succinctly, "Sometime ago a book entitled, *I Prayed Myself Slim!* told the story of an obese 'Cinderella' who had been trapped in her own body. In a fit of spirituality, she took her overweight condition to Christ, and He began to help her lose weight. Overnight, she was transformed into a beautiful princess, desired by the most exciting bachelors in town. God had rescued her from her fate as a wallflower and cast her gloriously into the fast lane of life! Naturally, she gave all the credit to God. Perhaps the young lady should have asked, 'Does God want the credit?'

"God does want us to glorify His Son and to escape the prison of self. Yet, a new Christian egotism insists that a Christianized self is an adequate center for life."[3]

Within the Western world there is a commercial segment that uses Christianity as a front. One major marketing scheme uses Biblical phrases and ideas to promote its own brand of egoism, wealth, and power. In his revealing book, *Fake It Till You Make It,* Phil Kerns tells of a sales rally where a leading distributor was telling how God established the marketing plan for Moses.

> And Moses shrugged and God began to describe the promised land, 'And here's how you'll get there,' and a white board mysteriously appeared behind God. He took a magic marker, and He drew a great big circle on the board and said, 'Moses, this is you' and drew a line with a circle at the top and said, 'I AM YOUR SPONSOR!'[4]

Besides this type of blasphemous trivia, there is a concept that says if you "dream" and "fake it till you make it," you can do anything. It is the power of positive thinking which teaches that you can do anything and everything, the powers are within you, and you need no other power because of your "innate" potential.

As a result of this fuzzy, egocentric reasoning, many Christians are unsure of what happens to people when they die. The concept that man does not really die at death but enters some mystical spirit world either for punishment or reward is compatible with the Hindu concept of reincarnation. The Monistic view of the self-help movement teaches that man somehow is in contact with "universal power" and beings. Therefore, man never really dies, but transfers from one level of "being" or "energy" to another. Without a firm base within the Holy Scriptures, many Christians are vulnerable to "supranormal" experiences. The Bible clearly states, "For the living know that they will die, but the dead know nothing; they have no further reward, and even the memory of them is forgotten."[5] If we would but cling to the objective demonstration of universal order as depicted in Scripture, we would be less susceptible to Satan's trap.

Jesus Christ came to this earth for one purpose and that was to heal a broken relationship between His people and Himself. The question is not what I can do, but what can I be through the power of God?

> His divine power has given us everything we need for life and godliness through our knowledge of Him who called us by His own glory and goodness. Through these He has given us His very great and precious promises, so that through them you may participate in the divine nature and escape the corruption in the world caused by evil desires.[6]

"All have sinned and come short of the glory of God."[7] All are separated from God by sin until a choice is made to re-establish that connection with God. The absence of something to DO to merit this gift strikes at the heart of the self-help movement. It shatters egocentric methodology and crumbles human pride. To remain true to its name, Christianity must then divorce itself from everything that smacks of humanism, the worship of the innate power of man. Instead, God now supplies the power for change in the life. There is a Creator-creature posture that bears the fruit of love, self-control and a willingness to be what God designs.

> But who are you, O man, to talk back to God? Shall what is formed say to him who formed it,'Why did you make me like this?' Does not the potter have the right to make out of the same lump of clay some pottery for noble purposes and some for common use?[8]

Until the Christian learns this, he makes himself less responsive to the drawing power of God by trying to do everything his own way. "Saving" people from heart disease, smoking and alcohol with techniques designed by Satan, will make the children of men less open to the power of the Gospel of Jesus Christ! Yes, healthy, but eternally lost.

Chapter Twelve

PUTTING IT ALL TOGETHER

> None are in greater danger from the influence of evil spirits than those who, notwithstanding the direct and ample testimony of the Scriptures, deny the existence and agency of the Devil and his angels. So long as we are ignorant of their wiles, they have almost inconceivable advantage; many give heed to their suggestions while they suppose themselves to be following the dictates of their own wisdom.... There is nothing the great deceiver fears so much as that we shall be acquainted with his devices.[1]

Some have soothingly stated that time and energy should not be devoted to looking at the "counterfeit." "If only the truth is told, the evil will take care of itself," they say. When I hear of ministers of the Gospel practicing iridology and find Christians being taught the occult art of behavioral kinesiology and mystical reflexology, it is time to do more than "teach the truth." It is time for a warning to be given. We are gullible, immature in the Word, and uninformed on God's true plan of health. Vaguely we recall that "drugs are bad" and "natural is better." With minds befogged by intemperate habits and unbridled passions, we reach out for something that is "holistic" and quick, some new herbal potion or a homeopathic tincture that will quickly change "energy," and perhaps we will not have to change our way of life. Our carnal, pride-filled nature loves to be titillated with the idea of increasing our personal "potential" and sense of "control" by thinking only positive thoughts and "visualizing" self as a good person without any recognition of our truly despicable state and of the power of God to change the human heart.

In the Old Testament, the prophets of God pointed out the pitfalls of heathen and occult practices.

> When you enter the land the Lord your God is giving you, do not learn to imitate the detestable ways of the nations there. Let no one be found among you who.... practices divination or sorcery, interprets omens, engages in witchcraft, or casts spells, or who is a medium or spiritist or who consults the dead. Anyone who does these things is detestable to the Lord, and because of these detestable practices the Lord your God will drive out those nations before you. You must be blameless before the Lord your God.[2]

One Christian writer decried the "holistic health" movement of the mid-nineteenth century.

> Thousands.... have been spoiled through the philosophy of phrenology and animal magnetism, and have been driven into infidelity.... Some will be tempted to receive these wonders as from God. The sick will be healed before us. Miracles will be performed in our sight. Are we prepared for the trial which awaits us when the lying wonders of Satan shall be more fully exhibited?.... We must all now seek to arm ourselves for the contest in which we must soon engage. Faith in God's Word, prayerfully studied and practically applied, will be our shield from Satan's power and will bring us off conquerors through the blood of Christ.[3]

These warnings are relevant now. The same holistic healing methods and techniques are being used today. Animal magnetism was originally based on the study of astrology. Mesmerism was very similar to the modern touch therapies and kinesiology. Reading auras and applying acupuncture and reflexology deal with the "electric currents." Iridology is similar to phrenology. The "human potential" movement is no different than the "mind sciences" of yesteryear.

> If Satan can so befog and deceive the human mind as to lead mortals to think that there is an inherent power in themselves to accomplish great and good works, they cease to rely upon God to do for them that which they think there is power in themselves to do.[4]

The consequences of dabbling in these areas may have far-reaching and eternal consequences. No longer can a person join himself to an advisor or healer without first knowing the healer's world view. Unknowingly, he may be opening himself to the occult. Demon possession is the result of using the older mystical healing methods of one hundred years ago.

> Satan often finds a powerful agency for evil in the power which one human mind is capable of exerting on another human mind.... Often in the day of His earthly ministry, the Saviour met His adversary in human form, when Satan, as an unclean spirit took possession of men. Satan takes possession of the minds of men today.... While men are spiritually sleeping, the enemy accomplishes his work of iniquity.[5]

Let us now summarize the common characteristics of holistic health.

ENERGY: This is a recurring theme. It may be called many things. The Hindus call it "Prana." Taoism and ancient Chinese medicine call it "Chi," "Ki" or "Qi." D.D. Palmer, the founder of chiropractics, called the same energy "The Innate." Franz Anton Mesmer used the word "Animal Magnetism" and the witch doctors of Polynesia refer to "Mana." Parapsychologists call it "Bioplasma." George Lucas of Star Wars fame calls it "The Force." But, by whatever name, they are all "Satan's electric currents." Beware of techniques that are stated to balance or increase energies or vibrations.

WORLD VIEW: Monism or Pantheism predominates the philosophy of the holistic healers. You are promised to become part of the "cosmic whole," the "Christ-self." In essence, you can become your own god. No matter how appealing this may sound, it is far from the truth. Unity of the whole world may be a lofty goal, but it will not happen without Jesus Christ as the Saviour.

AFTER DEATH: Reincarnation is a recurring theme. Some form of life after death in varying spiritual or physical forms must be included in holistic health teaching to answer the metaphysical questions inherent in mankind. The Scriptures clearly refute incarnation. (Eccl. 9:5, Job 3:11, 1 Thess. 4:13–18)

SEMANTICS: Watch the words closely. They may not mean what you think they do. Here is a simple "New Thought" glossary that may have some minor variations from technique to technique.

1. The Christ: Individualized in humanity, the perfect human in each of us, with Jesus Christ of Nazareth being only one example of "Christ."

2. Death: An illusion, the deception of a false belief. Since humanity's true nature is the mind which partakes of the "Mind of God," there is no death. Death is merely an occasion for spiritual advancement.

3. Disease: A disturbance in the inner spiritual body that is causally manifested in the outer, physical body. The source of disturbance is attributed to such things as false belief, wrong thinking, or ignorance of our true nature. This is in marked contrast to the cause and effect relationship of disease as seen in the various sciences such as bacteriology.

4. God: Although spoken of in personal terms, God is primarily considered an impersonal principle. God is First Cause, Substance, Mind Spirit, Life Principle, the Ultimate Essence behind all things. The universe is the body of God, the thought of God made manifest.

5. Humanity: Each person is an individualization of the Infinite Spirit of God, an incarnation of the Divine Mind. Although God's being and humanity's differ in degree, they are identical in essence.

6. Salvation: The realization of one's divine nature and perfect self Salvation depends not on personal faith in the sacrificial death of Jesus Christ, but on knowledge of our real nature and appropriate use of spiritual laws (right thinking). Salvation is universal, since it is the end to which all people move in the process of spiritual progression.

7. Sin: The separation from God, which is normally seen as a definition of sin, is here seen as a false belief. Such an error of the mind gives reality to evil, disease, and death, and darkens the ability to see one's true self as an individualization of the "Mind of God."

8. Pseudoscientific: There will always be some form of explanation of how something works. The explanation will often be couched in scientific terms that may sound somewhat plausible. Take this example from Irving Oyle's book entitled, *Time, Space, and the Mind* as quoted in "The Holistic Healers": "The idea of the identity of energy and matter has enormous implications for all the healing professions. It gives us a theoretical basis from which to consider therapeutic methods such as acupuncture, which purport to restore normal bodily states by manipulating the flow of cosmic energy. If energy and matter are indeed complementary states of a single entity, perhaps it is not unreasonable to hypothesize that by attention to the energy level, we can effect changes in the matter of the physical body."[6] What was said? It doesn't really make much difference as long as it sounds scientific and convinces you that this is a modern thought that deserves your confidence.

Naively, many Christians have thought that anything that helps someone is "good" and obviously from God. This assumption is based on ignorance of the Scriptures which clearly state,

> The coming of the lawless one will be in accordance with the work of Satan displayed in all kinds of counterfeit miracles, signs and wonders, and in every sort of evil that deceives those who are perishing. They perish because they refused to love the truth and so be saved.[7]

Thus Satan uses good events with false methods to deceive. What criteria can be used to discern between true and false?

1. Where did it come from? In other words, what is its source? Does it have mystical roots? What did the founder believe? What was his life story?

2. What company does the technique keep? Who uses it and what other therapies are included?

3. What is the ultimate direction that the therapy is headed? Am I led toward Jesus Christ or away from Him? Do I still need Him as a Saviour? Or have I become my own saviour?

4. Does it follow the known laws of physiology? It is very important to study the physiology or methods of action that have been delineated by those not involved in the therapy itself. The explanation given by the one pushing his technique, who profits from the product or method, is rarely reliable. There are some very convincing explanations of "toxins," "blockers," and "deficiencies" that in the light of pure physiology have little or no meaning.

5. Who receives the credit for the healing: the technique, or God? These definitions and criteria can serve to guide the "honest seeker of truth." There are a multitude of additional holistic health techniques which must receive your evaluation before allowing them to be used in your behalf.

> I entreat that there may be a putting away from the life every action which does not bear the approval of God. We are drawing near to the close of earth's history; the battle is growing daily more fierce.[8]

This is no time for casual dabbling in "arts" that could lead the individual into spiritually destructive practices. The next chapter will introduce a safe plan of health that each individual may participate in freely.

Chapter Thirteen

LIFESTYLE FOR HEALTH AND HEALING

What's left? It seems as if traditional, orthodox medicine has betrayed our confidence in its mechanical nonhuman way. The alternative therapies have strange roots of demonic origin despite the more "balanced" approach to the human being. Where can I turn for help? What is "truth"? The reader is invited to thoughtfully consider the following plan for optimal health.

TRUST IN GOD: The immune system is the bulwark against disease. God placed this complex, poorly understood organ system in our bodies to protect us from being invaded by the harsh environment He knew we would live in. This system is designed to protect us against everything from cancer to the common cold. It differentiates between the proteins of our body and the proteins of the foods we eat and other substances that we contact. The components of the immune system include the spleen, bone marrow, thymus gland, lymph channels, and multiple deposits of lymphoid tissue throughout the body. It is intricately intertwined with the other organ systems, even the mind.

Christopher W. Stout and Larry J. Bloom at the University of Colorado have shown that the nervous, uptight student is much more susceptible to colds.[1] Even blood levels of cholesterol are increased by stress within the mind.[2] Bernard Linn of the University of Miami found that the white blood count was depressed during the grieving period of those who had lost a spouse in death.[3] Guilt is a form of separation similar to the grieving time. Our sins or rebellion against God cause a definite sense of separation from His power and presence. It is possible that the immune system can be depressed by guilt. This should come as no surprise, as David recorded in the book of Psalms his own experience of a depressed immune system. "When I kept silent, my bones wasted away through my groaning all day long."[4] "Because of your wrath there is no health in my body; my bones have no soundness because of my sin. My guilt has overwhelmed me like a burden too heavy to bear. My wounds fester and are loathsome…. my back is filled with searing pain;…. my sighing is not hidden from you. My heart pounds, my strength fails me; even the light has gone from my eyes."[5] David was suffering from the consequences of guilt. Scientists today tell us that this is the most powerful negative emotion that we can experience.[6] To treat disease or maintain optimal health, our immune system must be functioning well. To know that Jesus Christ died to do away with my guilt and to provide the power to overcome sin is the most important health information that I can have and experience. No one has expressed this joy of well-being better than David.

> Let me hear joy and gladness; let the bones you have crushed rejoice…. Create in me a pure heart, O God, and renew a steadfast spirit within me…. Restore to me the joy of your salvation and grant me a willing spirit, to sustain me.[7]

> He lifted me out of the slimy pit, out of the mud and mire; he set my feet on a rock and gave me a firm place to stand. He put a new song in my mouth, a hymn of praise to our God. Many will see and fear and put their trust in the Lord.[8]

I believe Christians have health information available to them which could revolutionize medical therapy. When we learn to trust fully in God's healing methods, we can have optimum physical, mental and spiritual health.

SUNLIGHT: The sun is taken for granted. We use it more as a marker for day and night and forget that it has many health-giving properties, both maintenance and remedial. The ultraviolet rays are active in the reduction of harmful bacteria[9] and can even help in the control of body weight.[10] Sunlight has much to do with the delicate balance of our sex hormones,[11] and even transforms cholesterol into Vitamin D, thus contributing to the control of calcium and phosphorous in the body.[12] These and many other physiological functions that are still not identified by science, lead to a sense of well-being when we are out in the sunshine. If a person is ill, acutely or chronically, it is vital that each day he or she receive a "dose" of sunshine. There is no charge for this service. God has made it available to all.

WATER: Despite our somewhat "solid" appearance, our bodies are 70% water. The precious fluids of the body are economically preserved by a recirculation system that only our efficient Creator God could have designed. Without this system we would teeter between drowning and desiccation. But still some water must be added each day to the system to replace the losses through breathing, sweating and elimination. It is surprising how many of us refuse to drink those simple seven or eight glasses of water daily. Some seem to think of water as a poison. If we had to pay a large price for it, or could get it only at some exotic health food store, perhaps we would use it more readily. Until we are thoroughly rehydrated, our thirst can not be trusted to guide us. It may be necessary to measure out adequate amounts of water and then make sure that we drink that amount in any 24 hour period of time.

Cold water quenches what thirst we do have before we have had time to drink an adequate amount. The stomach then has to warm ice water to body temperature, thereby using valuable energy. Drinking water with our meals is not best because it dilutes the digestive enzymes and also makes us able to swallow food before it has been well chewed and mixed with the salivary enzymes that start the digestive process.

Water is useful externally as well. Going far beyond cleanliness, hydrotherapy or water therapy can be a simple remedy for the ill. Water therapy is not a speedy method, but instead takes patience, gentleness, and kindness to apply. The physiological principles can be taken from the book *Home Remedies* by Drs. Agatha and Calvin Thrash. Colds, flu, menstrual cramps, and headaches respond well to the application of water.[13] In more serious infectious diseases, hydrotherapy can be a useful assistance. Physical therapists are beginning to use more cryotherapy, or cold therapy, for a variety of injuries and inflammatory problems such as arthritis.[14]

Water, though a relatively simple agent, was not developed in some laboratory. Man can take no credit for this most amazing substance, but he can take the responsibility to use it wisely.

TEMPERANCE: This word means the avoidance of harmful substances and practices, and the moderate or wise use of that which is helpful. Think what would happen to the incidence of lung cancer if we, by some miracle, could do away with tobacco. Cirrhosis of the liver would become a rarity if we did not use alcohol as a beverage. Gonorrhea, AIDS, and other sexually transmitted diseases would disappear if men and women would be satisfied with God's plan for sexual fulfillment.

As we look at the areas of not only heart disease but also cancer of the breast and colon, we see obesity as one of the leading risk factors. Adult onset diabetes, which costs America $13.5 billion annually,[15] would become a rare disease if there was a change in lifestyle.

Controlling our lives seems impossible at times. Trying harder doesn't help. Fear of cancer, heart disease, disability or death will not change a habit permanently. There is only one answer.

> For the grace of God that brings salvation has appeared to all men. It teaches us to say 'No' to ungodliness and worldly passion, and to live self-controlled, upright and godly lives in this present age...[16]

AIR: You can't live long without it! But, just like the sunlight, we take it for granted. Today, pollution of our precious air envelope is taking place. Carbon monoxide, sulfur oxide, sulfates, nitrogen oxide, benzopyrene, ozone, cadmium and mercury are just a few of its many pollutants. Despite all this, polluted air is better than no air. Trees, greenery, and water will help with the purification of air and add beneficial negative ions. Dr. George Chen has summarized the effects of negative and positive ions:

> ...the small negatively charged air ions give a feeling of exhilaration and apparent improvement of health. Inhalation of positive ions results in headache, dizziness, nausea, and a feeling of fatigue. The positive ions increase the respiration rate, basal metabolism and blood pressure. Negative ions decrease these functions.[17]

Robles, Borrill and Medina repeatedly exposed 30 hypertensive patients for 25-minute sessions to negative air ionization. Twenty-four treated exclusively with this physical method showed an average reduction of systolic blood pressure of 39 mmHg.[18] Negative air ions affect the breathing mechanism by dilating the windpipe and causing the cilia lining it to move faster in order to make a more effective cleansing of the area....[19] Marked relief of hay fever symptoms was noted in two-thirds of the patients exposed to artificially ionized negative air....[20] "Even tumor growth, in one experiment, was decreased when exposed to negative ions."[21] It sounds almost too good to be true. But it is a fact, and we can take advantage of this gift from God.

NUTRITION: Everyone likes to talk about food. We are what we eat, and it is this fact that makes our diet so important for health. Conservative estimates are made that half of all cancers are related to our high fat, high sugar, low fiber and low nutrient diets.[22] Colon cancer and other gastrointestinal malignancies have been linked with diet.[23,24] Both obesity and elevated blood levels of cholesterol can increase the risk for breast cancer.[25] Consumption of foods that are high in vitamin A and other plant substances such as lignins[26] have been found to be higher in those who are free from cancer. These foods include the cabbage family, carrots and other yellow vegetables. It would be wise to include foods from this group in the daily dietary plan. By now everyone knows that there is a relationship between heart disease and the diet that we eat.[27] The real question is, has this knowledge made any difference in the lifestyle? Foods that are high in animal protein, fat and cholesterol make it more likely for a susceptible person to have coronary heart disease. The blood vessels to this critical organ of the body become clogged with fatty deposits, fibrous tissue, calcium and clotted blood. Since the only source of cholesterol outside of our own body is the animal products that we eat, the vegetarian diet offers the chance to avoid this risk factor. Many studies have shown that the process of atherosclerosis or hardening of the arteries can be reversed over a period of time by the use of a low cholesterol, vegetarian diet.[28]

REST: During the waking hours, our body concentrates on action and motion. Hormones such as epinephrine (adrenaline), cortisol and glycogen use up body proteins. No extra energy is used for the repair or replacement of worn-out parts. It is during the sleeping hours that this activity takes place. When we sleep, the hormonal balance shifts to an anabolic or "building" mode. Insulin, testosterone and other building hormones are set to work building new proteins for the body.[29] Sleep is of more value than just something to do when you are too tired to work any more. It is a time of preparation for another day. Muscle tissue, blood components and even bones are made during these precious hours of rest and sleep. It would be wise if we would use the Biblical demarcation of time, "evening and morning were the first day." Planning well for the next day does not begin at six o'clock in the morning. It begins the night before by getting to bed on time.

Paul has some wise counsel for us and our Hebrew friends.

> Therefore, since the promise of entering His rest still stands, let us be careful that none of you be found to have fallen short of it.... There remains, then, a Sabbath-rest for the

people of God; for anyone who enters God's rest also rests from his own work, just as God did from His.[30]

EXERCISE: "Use it or lose it." This slogan applies directly to our bodies. God created the body for action, and without it immediate decay begins. If you have ever had an arm or a leg in a cast for any period of time, you know it is not long before the muscle tissue begins to shrink and become weak. It is not just muscles that get weak with the lack of exercise; even the bones get weak.[31] Osteoporosis, or loss of mineral content of the bones, is partially caused by inactivity. Exercise may be as important in the prevention of this dreaded disease as the amount of calcium consumed in the diet.

For those who want to lose weight we might say, "If you don't use it, you won't lose it." Exercise forms the basis of any sound weight-control program. Without this stimulant of metabolism, dietary restrictions to lose weight will be stringent in that the whole metabolism is "on famine alert" and very little of this weight loss is permanent. Exercise also assists with the self-image and psychological aspects of weight control.[32]

Vigorous sustained exercise aids in the maintenance or repair of the heart. This is accomplished by decreasing the blood pressure and the heart rate, increasing the uptake of oxygen and altering the blood lipids.[33] With all of these advantages of exercise, it seems it would need no further support. But, there is more. Exercise is also a major feature in stress management programs. Special "well-being" hormones are released within the mind during vigorous exercise. Perhaps you have felt the peacefulness of mind that comes during or after a good physical workout.

These eight principles of good health form a plan that God has ordained to preserve health and treat disease. They seem so self-evident that we might, at first glance, think that they are too unsophisticated to compete with modern-day heart transplants and kidney dialysis machines. But, hopefully, the scientific corroboration of these principles will convince you that they are worth the time and the effort to institute them into your own lifestyle. Medical wisdom has always known that prevention is much better than cure. The lifestyle measures that you have just reviewed could have a strong impact against the staggering incidence of heart disease, cancer, hypertension, and stroke that have paralyzed the Western world and now even threaten other countries of the world that have adopted the Western lifestyle of high stress, low exercise, and over-nutrition. Even for those that already suffer from these degenerative diseases, there is the hope of renewal and healing through the use of the lifestyle measures. As simple as it sounds, this could save the lives of millions of people. It is up to you to practice and promote good health for yourself and those within your sphere of influence. Join me today in a lifestyle that brings health and healing.

REFERENCES

Chapter 1: The Revelation

1. 2 Thessalonians 2:9–10, NIV.
2. White, E.G., *Early Writings,* (Washington, D.C.: Review and Herald Publishing Association, 1882, 1945), p. 191.

Chapter 2: The Way is Prepared

1. Revelation 11:3, 7, NIV.
2. Scott, *Life of Napoleon,* Vol. I, Ch. 17.
3. "Blackwood's Magazine," November 1870
4. Feruson, W., *A Survey of European Civilization,* (Boston: 3rd Edition, Houghton Mifflin Co.), p. 578.
5. *Ibid.,* P. 582–584.
6. Robinson, Victor, *The Story of Medicine,* (New York: Tudor Publishing Co.), p. 347.
7. *Ibid.,* p. 348.
8. Garrison, Fielding H., *An Introduction to the History of Medicine,* (Philadelphia: W.B. Saunders Co.), p. 427.
9. *Ibid.,* p. 428.
10. White, E. G., *Testimonies,* Vol. I, (Mountain View, California: Pacific Press Publishing Association, 1948), p.297.
11. *Ibid.,* p. 209.

Chapter 3: The New Age Success

1. Jonah 1:6, NIV.
2. Fetcho, David, *"In the Face of the Tempest, Jonah Sleeps,"* SPC JOURNAL, (August, 1978), p. 4.
3. Tillich, Paul, *The Shaking of the Foundation,* (Pelican edition, 1962). p. 63.

4. Robinson, John A. T., *Honest to God,* (Philadelphia: The Westminster Press, 1963), p. 51.
5. *Ibid.,* p. 58.
6. "The Graduate Review," November 1976, p. 3.
7. *Ibid.,* p. 4.
8. Doshin, *The Essentials of Zen Buddhism,* p. 127.
9. Fetcho, *op. cit.* p. 3.

Chapter 4: The Techniques

1. White, E. G., *Testimonies,* Vol. V, *op.cit.* pp. 192–193.
2. Kul, Djwal, *Intermediate Studies of the Human Aura,* (Los Angeles: Summit University Press, 1980), p. 1.
3. Hill, Ann, A *Visual Encyclopedia of Unconventional Medicine,* (New York: Crown Publishers, Inc., 1979), p. 46.
4. Kul, *op. cit.* p. 79.
5. *Ibid.,* plate 19.
6. Hill, *op. cit.* p. 219.

Chapter 5: The Pendulum and Stick

1. Weldon, John, *Psychic Healing,* (Chicago: Moody Press, 1982) pp. 60–62. Quoting from *Theosophical Research Center Mystery of Healing,* (Theosophical Publishing House, 1958), pp. 63–65.
2. Hill, *op. cit.* p. 171.
3. Hahnemann, Samuel, *Organon of Medicine,* (New Delhi: B. Jain Publishers, 1980, p. 56.
4. Hill, *op. cit.* p. 161.
5. *Ibid.,* p. 164.
6. Leftwich, Robert, *Dowsing—the Ancient Art Rhabdomancy,* (New York: Samuel Weiser, Inc., 1976), p. 9.
7. *Ibid.,* pp. 23–24.
8. *Ibid.,* P. 33.
9. Hester, Ben, *Dowsing—An Expose of Hidden Occult Forces,* (Yucaipa, California: U. S. Business Specialties, 1982), p. 129.
10. Private letter made available to the author.
11. *Ibid.*

12. Hester, Ben, *The Paradise Valley Sanitarium "Miracle Well" as the Justification of Dowsing,* (Gerald Rentfro, 11845 S. Mt. Vernon Ave, Colton, Calif 92324), p. 7.
13. Hosea 4:12. NIV.
14. Revelation 16:12–16. NIV.

Chapter 6: Acupuncture and Reflexology

1. Hill, *op. cit.* p. 57.
2. "Symposium: Acupuncture Anesthesia," *Anesthesiology Review,* June, 1974, p. 17.
3. John de Romanett, *Acupuncture, Mesmerism and Hypnotism,* (Wenatchee, Wa.: Audiotronics of Wenatchee, 1975), p. 9.
4. Weldon, John and Wilson, Clifford, *Occult Shock and Psychic Forces,* (San Diego, Master Books, 1980), pp. 193–194.
5. 1 Samuel 28:3, NIV.
6. *Ibid.,* 28:4.
7. Deuteronomy 18:10–12, NIV.

Chapter 7: Applied and Behavioral Kenesiology

1. Wilson and Weldon, *op. cit.* p. 190.
2. Hill, *op. cit.* p. 44.
3. Dimond, John, *Your Body doesn't Lie,* (New York: Warner Books, 1979), p. 197.
4. *Ibid.,* p. 61.
5. Kul, *op. cit.* plate 3.

Chapter 8: Iridology

1. Psalm 38:10, NIV.
2. Simon, Allies et al. "An Evaluation of Iridology." *Journal of the American Medical Association,* pp. 242:1380–1389.
3. "What Your Eyes Tell You About Your Health," *Esquire,* January, 1978.
4. Oakley, E. M., "Your Eyes Reflect Your Health," *New Realities,* Vol. I, No. 3, p. 50.
5. Koch, Kurt, *The Devil's Alphabet,* p. 38, 39.
6. Maxwell, Jessica, *The Eye-Body Connection,* (New York: Warner Books, 1980), p. 5.
7. Kul, *op. cit.,* plate 4.

8. Collyer, Robert H., *Psychography, or the Embodiment of Thought: With an Analysis of PhrenoMagnetism, Neurology and Mental Hallucination, Including Rules to Govern and Produce the Magnetic State,* (Philadelphia: Zieber and Co., 1843), p. 19.
9. Hacket, Willis, *Moulding the Christian Mind,* p. 28.
10. White, E. G., *Testimonies,* Vol. I, *op. cit.,* p. 290.
11. 2 Thessalonians 2:9, 10, NIV.
12. Revelation 18:4, NIV.

Chapter 9: Herbal Therapy

1. Revelation 22:1, 2, NIV.
2. Virgil, *Aeneid XII,* p. 412.
3. Tyler, *The Honest Herbal,* (Philadelphia, PA: George F. Stickley Co.), p. 7.
4. Hill, *op. cit.,* p. 12.
5. White, E. G., *Selected Messages,* Vol. II, (Washington, D. C.: Review and Herald Publishing Association, 1958), p. 295.
6. *Ibid., 294.*
7. White, E. G., *Spiritual Gifts,* Vol. IV, (Battle Creek, Michigan: Steamboat Press, 1864), p. 140.
8. Tyler, *op. cit.* p. 175.

Chapter 10: Roots of Healing Methods

1. Hahnemenn, *op. cit.,* p. 215.
2. Hill, *op. cit.,* p. 23.
3. Wilson and Weldon, *op. cit.,* pp. 234–235.
4. White, E. G., *Selected Messages,* Vol. II, *op. cit.,* p. 282.
5. Wilson and Weldon, *op. cit.,* p. 235.
6. *Ibid.,* p. 209.
7. *Ibid.,* p. 215.
8. Ernest H. J. Steed, *Two Be One,* (Plainfield, New Jersey: Logos International, 1978), p. 89.
9. *Ibid.,* p. 95.
10. White, E. G., Testimonies, Vol. V, op. *cit.,* p. 443.

Chapter 11: Self-Help

1. White, John, "What is Enlightenment?" *New Realities,* (March/April 1985) p. 56.
2. *Ibid.,* p. 56, 57.
3. Miller, Calvin, "Family Life Today," *Invitation to Intimacy,* (May/June 1985), p. 27.
4. Kerns, Phil, *Fake It Til You Make It!* (Carlton, Oregon: Victory Press, 1982), p. 49.
5. Ecclesiastes 9:5. NIV.
6. 2 Peter 1:3, 4. NIV.
7. Romans 3:23. *NW.*
8. Romans 9:20, 21. NIV.

Chapter 12: Putting It AR Together

1. White, E. G., *The Great Controversy,* (Mountain View, California, 1950) p. 516.
2. Deuteronomy 18:9)13. NIV.
3. White, E. G., *Testimonies,* Vol. I, *op. cit.* pp. 297, 302.
4. *Ibid.,* p. 294.
5. White, E. G., *Selected Messages,* Vol. II, *op. cit.* pp. 353, 354.
6. Reisser, Paul C., Reisser, Teri K., and Weldon, John, *The Holistic Healers,* (Downers Grove, Illinois: Inter Varsity Press, 1983), p. 36.
7. 2 Thessalonians 2:9–10. NIV.
8. White, E. G., *Selected Messages,* Vol. II, *op. cit.* p. 353.

Chapter 13: Lifestyle For Health, Prevention And Treatment

1. Stout, C., and Bloom, L., "Type A Behavior and Upper Respiratory Infections," *Journal of :Iuman Stress,* (June 1982), pp. 4–7.
2. van Dooren, L., and Orlebke, K.F., "Stress, Personality and Serum Cholesterol Level," *Journal of Human Stress,* (December 1982), pp. 24–29.
3. Martin, J., "Of Mind and Morbidity: Can Stress and Grief Depress Immunity?," *Journal of the American Medical Association,* 248:405–407, 1982.

4. Psalm 32:8. NIV.
5. Ibid., 38:3–10. NIV.
6. Lynch, James J., *The Broken Heart*, (New York: Basic Books, Inc. Publishers, 1979), p. 41.
7. Psalm 51:8)12. NIV.
8. *Ibid.*, 40:2–3. NIV.
9. Moggio, M., Goldner, L., and McCullian, D., "Wound Infections in Patients Undergoing Total Hip Arthroplasty," ARCH SURG, 114:815–823, 1979.
10. Ellinger, F., "The Influence of Ultraviolet Rays on the Body Weight," *Radiology*, 32:157, 1939.
11. Allen, R. M., Cureton, T. K., "Effect of Ultraviolet Radiation on Physical Fitness," *Archives of Physical Medicine*, 26:641–644, 1945.
12. Rauschkolb, E. W., Farrell, G., Knox, J. M., "Effects of Ultraviolet Light on Skin Cholesterol," *Journal of Invest. Derm.*, 49:632–636, 1967.
13. Thrash, A., and Thrash, C., *Home Remedies*, (Seale, Alabama: Uchee Pines Institute, 1981).
14. Bengston, R., Warfield, C., "Physical Therapy for Pain Relief," *Hospital Practices*, (August 1984), p. 84.
15. *Diabetes Dateline 6:1* (Sept/October 1985).
16. Titus 2:11–12. NIV.
17. Dessauer, F., Jahre, Z., "Forschung auf dem Physikalisch Medizinischen Grenzgebiet," *Georg Theime Leipez*, 1931.
18. Gorriti, A. R., Medina, A., "The Application of Ion Therapy in Hypertension Released," *the National Ministry of Public Health*, Buenos Aires, April 12, 1954.
19. Kreger, A. P., Smith, R. F., *Journal of General Physiology*, 43:533, 1960.
20. Komblueh, I. H., Griffin, J. E., "Artificial Air Ionization in Physical Medicine," *AM. J. PHY MED*, 34:618.
21. Eddy, W. H., "The Effect of Negative Ionization on Transplanted Tumors," *Cancer Research*, 11:245, 1951.
22. "Diet, Nutrition, and Cancer." National Research Council, Washington D. C.: *National Academy Press*, 1982.
23. Nair, P.P., "Diet, Nutrition Intake, and Metabolism in Populations at High and Low Risk for Colon Cancer," *Amer. J. Clin. Nut.*, 40:947–948, 1984.

24. Cummings, J. H., "Dietary Factors in the Aetiology of Gastrointestinal Cancer," *J. Hum. Nut.* 32:455–465, 1978.
25. Tartter, P.I., Aufses, A. H., "Cholesterol and Obesity as Prognostic Factors in Breast Cancer," *Cancer* 47:2222–2227, 1981.
26. Adlercreutz, H., Gorbach, S. L., "Excretion of the Lignins Enterolactone Enterodiol and of Equol in Omnivorous and Vegetarian Postmenopausal Women and in Women with Breast Cancer," *The Lancet* (Dec. 11, 1982) p. 1295–1298.
27. "Diet, Nutrition, and Cancer," (Washington, D.C.: *National Academy Press,* 1982), p. 14.
28. Daoud, A. S., Lee, K. T., "Regression of Advanced Atherosclerosis in Swine," *Arch Pathol Lab Med* 100:372–379.
29. Adam, K., Oswald, I., "Sleep Helps Healing," *Brit. Med. J.* 289:1400–1401, 1984.
30. Hebrews 4:1, 9. NIV.
31. Peck. W. A., "Osteoporosis," *Journal of the American Medical Association* 252:799–802, 1984.
32. Short, M. A., Pavlou, K., "Effects of Physical Conditioning on Self-concept Adult Obese Males," *Physical Therapy* 64:194–198.
33. Smith, R. J., "Physician-supervised Exercise Programs in Rehabilitation of Patients with Coronary Heart Disease," *JAMA* 245:1463–1466, 1981.

Other books by TEACH Services, Inc.

Absolutely Vegetarian   *Lorine Tadej* .... $ 8.95
A complete guide to maintaining a strict vegetarian lifestyle. A way to
reach your ideal weight and maintain it, as long as you live.

Adam's Table   *Reggi Burnett*........................... $ 8.95
A cookbook to help the user obtain optimum healthier and happier
lifestyle through changes in their cooking style. Originated from Adam's
Table Restaurant in Albuquerque, NM.

An Adventure in Cooking   *Joanne Chitwood Nowack*......... $12.95
This book has been compiled especially to teach young people, in a
step-by-step, progressive way, the art of vegetarian cookery. Cooking is
a real art, and very practical one too, since we need to eat every day.

The Art of Massage   *J. H. Kellogg* $12.95
A practical manual for the student, the nurse and the practitioner.

Caring Kitchen Recipes   *Gloria Lawson* $12.95
Specializes in recipes for better health that features: whole grains,
vegetarian, dairy-free and nourishing dessert recipes.

Don't Drink Your Milk   *Frank Oski, MD* .... $ 7.95
Dr. Oski, the head of Pediatrics at Johns Hopkins University School of
Medicine, gives the frightening new medical facts about the world's most
overrated nutrient.

Healing By God's Natural Methods   *Al. Wolfsen* .... $ 4.95
Al. Wolfsen has taught hundreds of sick people how to use only simple,
non-poisonous remedies.

Healthy Food Choices   *Leona R. Alderson* $14.95
Some special features include: guidelines for menu planning, breakfast
suggestions, ideas for brown bag lunches, and much more!

Hydrotherapy—Simple Treatments   *Thomas/Dail* .... $ 8.95
Help your body overcome common diseases using hydrotherapy and
simple home treatments.

Incredible Edibles   *Eriann Hullquist* .... $ 7.95
Some "health" meals taste bland, some are hard to make, others require
strange or hard to find ingredients. Eriann has developed a simple method
of meal preparation where each recipe looks good and tastes great.

Nature's Banquet   *Living Springs* $12.95
Cooking is an Art and a Science. You will find that the art and science
of cooking is especially enjoyable when using natural foods and when
learning to be a vegetarian cook. The art of food preparation will give
you the opportunity to exercise your enlightened preference and your
personality to create attractive, delicious and nutritious meals. The
science of cooking involves techniques and properties of food which
affect its successful preparation.

Nutrition Workshop Guide   *Eriann Hullquist* . . . . 10 for $ 9.95
Chock full of nutritional recipes, as well as lots of helpful nutritional tips
for special situations, such as road trips, fast foods, etc.

Protect Your Family Against AIDS   *J. & M. Wehr* . . . . $ 7.95
This book provides a detailed program used by those who have experienced good success against this deadly virus.

Quick-n-Easy Natural Recipes   *Lorrie Knutsen* . . . . $ 2.95
Every recipe has five or fewer ingredients and most take only minutes to
prepare. Now you can enjoy simple, natural recipes without the drudgery!

Returning Back To Eden   *Betty-Ann Peters* . . . . $ 9.95
These recipes have been taste-tested by the world-wide travelers that
have visited the Back to Eden Restaurant & Bakery in Minocqua, WI.

Stress: Taming the Tyrant   *Richard Neil*. . . . . $ 8.95
Stress is an inevitable part of our 20th century lifestyle. Under the proper
circumstances stress can be uplifting as well as depressing. It can either
help us grow our hasten or death. Find out how to control, manage and
modify stress.

375 Meatless Recipes–CENTURY 21   *Ethel Nelson, MD* . . . . . . $ 7.95
This book will help you learn how to feed your family in such a way that
they will enjoy eating the foods that nutritionists tell us are an absolute
must if we are going to make it into the twenty-first century.

Understanding the Body Organs   *Celeste Lee* . . . . $ 7.95
Simply and concisely explains how the body organs function and how
they relate to one another. Also includes the eight laws of health,
explaining each one and sharing many benefits that will be derived from
following the entire plan.

Who Killed Candida?   *Vicki Glassburn*. $17.95
Although diet is an important part of getting well, even the best food and
supplements are undermined if you continue to unknowingly support
yeast growth! The author will show you how making simple lifestyle
choices can actually STOP THE YEAST SUPPORT CYCLE that other
Candida programs do not address.

Whole Foods For Whole People *Lucy Fuller*. $10.95
Whole Foods For Whole People is not just a cookbook, but a manual to
teach people how they can live a longer, healthier lifestyle by using the
natural resources which surround us.

To order any of the above titles, see your local bookstore.

However, if you are unable to locate any title,
call 518/358-3652.